# ENDOMETRIOSIS DIET COOKBOOK

## FOR BEGINNERS

Healing Recipes to Manage Symptoms, Reduce Inflammation, and Boost Overall Well-Being

Kingsley Klopp

# *Table of Contents*

**Soups and Stew**

To show our appreciation for your purchase, we're delighted to offer you these special bonuses as a heartfelt thank you.

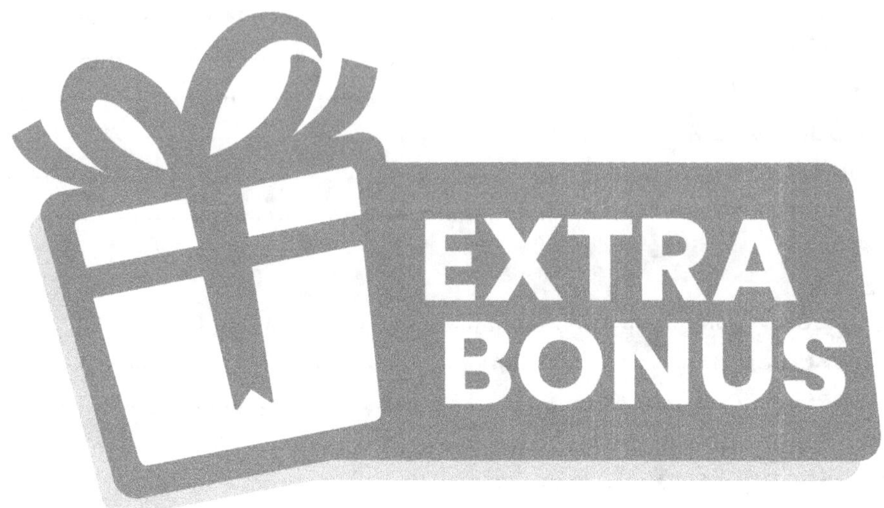


1. A Food Tracker Journal
2. Downloadable E-BOOK featuring full-color images of finished recipes

## A Note to Our Readers

We are thrilled to have you embark on this journey towards better health and well-being through the power of nutritious and delicious food. As you explore the recipes and tips within these pages, we want to share an important note with you. Each person's experience with endometriosis is unique, and so are their dietary needs. While this cookbook provides a variety of recipes designed to alleviate symptoms and promote overall health, it is crucial to recognize that individual responses to certain foods can vary. What works wonderfully for one person may not have the same effect for another. Therefore, we encourage you to listen to your body and make adjustments based on your personal needs and preferences.

If at any point you find yourself unsure about a particular recipe or ingredient, or if you have specific dietary concerns, please consult with your healthcare provider. Your doctor or a registered dietitian can offer personalized advice and ensure that your dietary choices are safe and effective for your unique situation. Their guidance is invaluable in tailoring a diet that supports your health and manages your symptoms effectively.

Additionally, while we have provided nutritional information for each recipe, please note that these figures are approximate. The actual nutritional content may vary depending on the specific brands and quantities of ingredients you use. For the most accurate nutritional information, we recommend using a nutritional calculator or app that allows you to input your exact ingredients.

Our goal is to empower you with knowledge and delicious recipes that can help manage your endometriosis symptoms and improve your quality of life. However, remember that this cookbook is a guide, not a one-size-fits-all solution. Your journey with endometriosis is personal, and your dietary choices should reflect your individual needs and circumstances.

Furthermore, If our cookbook has brought joy to your kitchen and table, we'd be thrilled to hear about your experiences in an Amazon review. On the flip side, if you stumble upon any hiccups while exploring our recipes, don't hesitate to get in touch at **kloppkingsley@gmail.com**. We're here to support your cooking journey every step of the way.

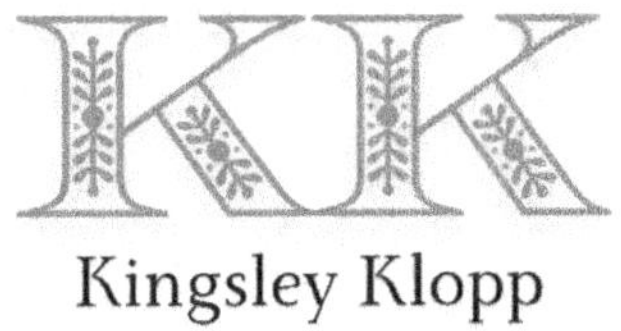

Kingsley Klopp

# Introduction

Endometriosis is a chronic, often debilitating condition that affects millions of women worldwide. For those living with this disease, daily life can be a constant battle against pain, fatigue, and emotional strain. The struggle is not only physical but also mental and emotional, as the persistent discomfort can impact every facet of life. Yet, amidst this challenge, there is a beacon of hope: the transformative power of diet. Welcome to the **Endometriosis Diet Cookbook for Beginners,** a carefully crafted guide designed to help you navigate the complexities of endometriosis through the healing power of food. This book is more than just a collection of recipes; it is a lifeline for those seeking relief and a sense of control over their health. By embracing the principles and recipes outlined in this book, you will embark on a journey toward improved well-being and a better quality of life. The connection between diet and endometriosis is profound. Scientific research and anecdotal evidence have consistently shown that certain foods can exacerbate endometriosis symptoms, while others can alleviate them. The right dietary choices can reduce inflammation, balance hormones, and strengthen the immune system, all of which play critical roles in managing endometriosis. This cookbook is rooted in these findings, offering a practical and delicious approach to dietary management. Understanding the challenges you face, this book is designed with empathy and practicality in mind. We recognize that the journey to dietary change can be daunting, especially when dealing with a chronic illness. Therefore, we have ensured that each recipe is not only nutritious but also easy to prepare and satisfying to eat. Whether you are a seasoned cook or a kitchen novice, you will find these recipes accessible and enjoyable.

The **Endometriosis Diet Cookbook for Beginners** is divided into several sections to guide you seamlessly through your dietary transformation. Starting with an informative overview of endometriosis and the role of diet in managing this condition, we provide you with the knowledge you need to make informed decisions. This is followed by practical tips on grocery shopping, meal planning, and cooking techniques that will become invaluable tools in your journey. Each recipe has been meticulously tested to ensure it meets the highest standards of nutrition and taste. From comforting breakfasts and hearty lunches to delicious dinners and snacks, every meal has been designed to support your health while tantalizing your taste buds. We have also included detailed nutritional information for each recipe, so you can track your intake and make adjustments as needed.

But this book is not just about food. It is about empowering you to take charge of your health and reclaim your life from the grip of endometriosis. Throughout the book, you will find inspiring stories from women who have successfully managed their symptoms through dietary changes. These stories serve as a testament to the potential of diet to bring about significant improvements in health and well-being. As you turn the pages of this cookbook, we hope you will feel a sense of hope and empowerment. Remember, every small change you make is a step towards a healthier, more vibrant you. Let this book be your guide, your companion, and your inspiration on this transformative journey. Welcome to the first step in reclaiming your health and living a life with less pain and more joy.

# Chapter 1: The Basics of the Endometriosis
## *What is Endometriosis?*

Endometriosis is a chronic, often painful condition that affects millions of women worldwide, yet it remains widely misunderstood and frequently misdiagnosed. Imagine waking up each day, knowing that you will face not only the usual challenges of life but also the relentless pain and discomfort that endometriosis brings. This is the reality for many women who live with this condition, which occurs when tissue similar to the lining inside the uterus, known as the endometrium, starts to grow outside the uterus. The name **"endometriosis"** might sound clinical and detached, but the experience is anything but. It's not just a medical term; it's a daily struggle that can significantly impact every aspect of a woman's life. These rogue endometrial-like tissues can be found on the ovaries, fallopian tubes, the outer surface of the uterus, and other organs within the pelvis. Each menstrual cycle, these tissues act as they would inside the uterus—thickening, breaking down, and bleeding. However, unlike the endometrial tissue within the uterus that exits the body during menstruation, this displaced tissue has no way to leave the body, causing inflammation, pain, and the formation of scar tissue.

For those suffering from endometriosis, the symptoms can be overwhelming. The most common symptom is pelvic pain, often associated with menstrual periods. But this isn't your typical menstrual cramp; the pain can be debilitating, sometimes described as stabbing or throbbing, and can persist throughout the month. Many women with endometriosis also experience severe menstrual bleeding, pain during intercourse, painful bowel movements or urination, and chronic fatigue. The physical pain is often accompanied by emotional distress, as the condition can lead to feelings of frustration, helplessness, and isolation. The journey to a diagnosis is often a long and arduous one. On average, it takes about seven years from the onset of symptoms for a woman to receive a correct diagnosis. This delay can be attributed to a lack of awareness about the condition among both women and healthcare providers, as well as the fact that the symptoms of endometriosis can mimic those of other conditions, such as irritable bowel syndrome (IBS) or pelvic inflammatory disease (PID).

Living with endometriosis can be incredibly isolating. The invisible nature of the illness means that others often cannot see the pain and suffering it causes, leading to misunderstandings and a lack of empathy. Women may feel pressured to downplay their symptoms to avoid being perceived as weak or overly dramatic. This stigma can prevent them from seeking the support they need and deserve. Endometriosis is not just a reproductive health issue; it's a whole-body issue that can affect a woman's physical, emotional, and social well-being. The chronic pain and fatigue can make it difficult to maintain employment, engage in social activities, or even perform everyday tasks. Relationships can also be strained, as partners may struggle to understand the severity of the condition and its impact on intimacy and daily life.

Despite the challenges, there is hope. Increased awareness and understanding of endometriosis are paving the way for better diagnosis and treatment options. Many women find relief through a combination of medical treatments, such as hormonal therapies and pain medications, and lifestyle changes, including diet and exercise. Support groups and counseling can also provide much-needed emotional support and a sense of community. In the end, it's essential to recognize that endometriosis is a significant health issue that deserves attention and empathy. By raising awareness and fostering a deeper understanding of the condition, we can help those affected by endometriosis feel seen, heard, and supported. It's a journey that no one should have to face alone, and with the right resources and compassion, we can make that journey a little easier.

# Understanding the Role of Diet in Managing Endometriosis

Understanding the role of diet in managing endometriosis is a powerful, hopeful journey that offers a glimmer of control over a condition often marked by pain and unpredictability. For many women, dietary changes can bring significant relief, transforming the way they experience life with endometriosis. Imagine finding solace in the foods you eat, discovering that what nourishes your body can also ease your suffering. This is the potential of a well-considered diet for endometriosis. Endometriosis is characterized by the growth of endometrial-like tissue outside the uterus, causing inflammation, pain, and the formation of scar tissue. While there is no cure for this chronic condition, diet can play a crucial role in managing symptoms and improving quality of life. The foods you choose to eat can either exacerbate inflammation and pain or help reduce them, making diet a critical component of holistic endometriosis care. The first step in understanding this dietary approach is recognizing the inflammatory nature of endometriosis. Inflammation is a key driver of the pain and discomfort associated with the condition. Therefore, focusing on an anti-inflammatory diet is essential. This means incorporating a variety of fresh fruits and vegetables, which are rich in antioxidants and can help combat oxidative stress and inflammation. Leafy greens, berries, and colorful vegetables are particularly beneficial. **Omega-3 fatty acids**, found in fatty fish like salmon, sardines, and mackerel, as well as in flaxseeds and walnuts, are known for their anti-inflammatory properties. Including these foods in your diet can help reduce inflammation and the severity of symptoms. On the other hand, it's important to limit the intake of omega-6 fatty acids, which are prevalent in processed and fried foods, as they can promote inflammation.

Another crucial aspect is the reduction of processed foods and sugars. These can contribute to inflammation and hormonal imbalances, exacerbating endometriosis symptoms. Instead, focus on whole grains, such as quinoa, brown rice, and oats, which provide sustained energy and support overall health without spiking blood sugar levels. Dairy and gluten are two food groups that some women with endometriosis find problematic. While not all women with endometriosis are sensitive to these foods, many report improvements in their symptoms when they eliminate or reduce dairy and gluten from their diets. Keeping a food diary can help identify any personal triggers and guide dietary adjustments.

Hydration also plays a significant role in managing endometriosis. Drinking plenty of water helps flush out toxins and supports overall bodily functions. Herbal teas, such as chamomile and ginger, can provide additional anti-inflammatory benefits and soothe digestive discomfort often associated with endometriosis. Lastly, it's essential to approach dietary changes with a mindset of self-care and compassion. Living with endometriosis can be an emotional rollercoaster, and making dietary changes can feel overwhelming. Remember that small, gradual changes are more sustainable and can lead to significant improvements over time. Seek support from nutritionists or dietitians who understand endometriosis, and connect with others who share similar experiences.

Incorporating these dietary principles into your life can empower you to take control of your health and alleviate some of the burdens of endometriosis. It's about more than just food; it's about reclaiming your well-being, finding comfort in nourishing meals, and nurturing your body with the respect and care it deserves.

# *Foods to Avoid*

**1. Processed and Refined Foods**

Processed and refined foods are often high in unhealthy fats, sugars, and additives that can increase inflammation in the body. These foods, such as packaged snacks, fast food, and sugary cereals, can contribute to hormonal imbalances and aggravate endometriosis symptoms. The high levels of trans fats found in many processed foods are particularly harmful, as they have been linked to increased inflammation and pain.

**2. Sugary Foods and Beverages**

Excessive sugar consumption can lead to increased levels of inflammation and insulin resistance. High insulin levels can disrupt hormonal balance, which is particularly detrimental for women with endometriosis. Avoiding sugary foods such as candies, pastries, sodas, and other sweetened beverages is essential. Instead, opt for natural sweeteners like honey or maple syrup in moderation, and prioritize whole fruits for a healthier source of sweetness.

**3. Red Meat and Processed Meats**

Red meat and processed meats, such as bacon, sausages, and deli meats, are associated with higher levels of prostaglandins, which can promote inflammation and pain. These meats also often contain hormones and antibiotics that can further disrupt the body's hormonal balance. It's beneficial to limit red meat consumption and choose lean proteins like poultry, fish, and plant-based sources such as beans and legumes.

**4. Dairy Products**

Dairy products can be problematic for some women with endometriosis. Dairy contains arachidonic acid, a fatty acid that can promote inflammation. Additionally, many dairy products contain hormones that can interfere with the body's natural hormonal balance. If dairy seems to worsen your symptoms, consider alternatives such as almond milk, coconut milk, or other plant-based milk products.

**5. Gluten**

Gluten is a protein found in wheat, barley, and rye. Some women with endometriosis find that gluten can trigger inflammation and exacerbate symptoms. While not everyone with endometriosis is sensitive to gluten, eliminating it from your diet may provide relief. Opt for gluten-free grains like quinoa, brown rice, and millet.

**6. Soy Products**

Soy contains phytoestrogens, which are plant compounds that mimic estrogen in the body. Since endometriosis is an estrogen-dependent condition, consuming large amounts of soy can potentially worsen symptoms. It's advisable to limit soy products such as tofu, soy milk, and edamame, especially if you notice that they trigger your symptoms.

**7. Caffeine and Alcohol**

Caffeine and alcohol can both have adverse effects on endometriosis. Caffeine can increase estrogen levels and lead to heightened pain, while alcohol can impair liver function, reducing its ability to process and eliminate excess hormones. Reducing or eliminating caffeine and alcohol from your diet can help manage symptoms more effectively. Opt for herbal teas and water to stay hydrated and support liver function.

**8. High-FODMAP Foods**

High-FODMAP foods can cause digestive issues, which are common in women with endometriosis. FODMAPs are short-chain carbohydrates that are poorly absorbed in the gut, leading to bloating, gas, and pain. Foods high in FODMAPs include onions, garlic, beans, and certain fruits like apples and pears. A low-FODMAP diet, under the guidance of a nutritionist, may help alleviate gastrointestinal symptoms.

Hence, avoiding these foods can play a significant role in managing endometriosis. It's important to listen to your body and note any foods that seem to trigger symptoms. Making dietary changes can be challenging, but the potential relief from pain and improvement in quality of life make it worthwhile. Always consider consulting with a healthcare provider or nutritionist to ensure that your diet is balanced and meets your nutritional needs while managing endometriosis.

# *Foods to Include*

## 1. Fruits and Vegetables

Fruits and vegetables are rich in vitamins, minerals, antioxidants, and fiber, making them essential for managing endometriosis. Antioxidants help combat oxidative stress and inflammation, which are key factors in endometriosis. Incorporate a variety of colorful fruits and vegetables to ensure a wide range of nutrients. Some particularly beneficial options include:

- **Leafy Greens:** Kale, spinach, and Swiss chard are high in antioxidants and anti-inflammatory compounds.
- **Berries:** Blueberries, strawberries, and raspberries are packed with antioxidants and vitamins.
- **Cruciferous Vegetables:** Broccoli, cauliflower, and Brussels sprouts contain compounds that support liver detoxification and hormone balance.
- **Citrus Fruits:** Oranges, lemons, and grapefruits are high in vitamin C, which boosts the immune system and reduces inflammation.

## 2. Whole Grains

Whole grains provide essential fiber, vitamins, and minerals that support digestive health and hormone balance. Fiber helps regulate blood sugar levels and promotes regular bowel movements, which is crucial for managing endometriosis symptoms. Include whole grains such as:

- **Quinoa:** A gluten-free grain high in protein and fiber.
- **Brown Rice:** A whole grain that provides sustained energy.
- **Oats:** Rich in fiber and helpful for maintaining stable blood sugar levels.
- **Millet:** A gluten-free grain that is easy to digest and nutritious.

## 3. Omega-3 Fatty Acids

Omega-3 fatty acids have powerful anti-inflammatory properties that can help reduce the severity of endometriosis symptoms. Include foods rich in omega-3s to support overall health:

- **Fatty Fish:** Salmon, mackerel, and sardines are excellent sources of omega-3s.
- **Chia Seeds:** High in omega-3s, fiber, and protein.
- **Flaxseeds:** Another great source of omega-3s; can be added to smoothies or oatmeal.
- **Walnuts:** Provide omega-3s and make for a healthy snack.

## 4. Lean Proteins

Lean proteins are important for maintaining muscle mass and overall health. They help keep you full and provide the building blocks for repairing tissues. Opt for lean proteins such as:

- **Chicken and Turkey:** Lean sources of protein that are easy to incorporate into meals.
- **Fish:** Besides being rich in omega-3s, fish provides high-quality protein.
- **Legumes:** Beans, lentils, and chickpeas are plant-based proteins that also offer fiber and essential nutrients.
- **Tofu and Tempeh:** Plant-based protein options that can be used in a variety of dishes.

## 5. Nuts and Seeds

Nuts and seeds are nutrient-dense foods that provide healthy fats, protein, and fiber. They are also rich in vitamins and minerals that support overall health:

- **Almonds:** High in healthy fats, protein, and magnesium.
- **Pumpkin Seeds:** A good source of zinc and magnesium, important for immune function and hormone balance.
- **Sunflower Seeds:** Rich in vitamin E, an antioxidant that helps reduce inflammation.

## 6. Healthy Fats

Healthy fats are essential for hormone production and reducing inflammation. Include sources of healthy fats such as:

- **Avocados:** High in monounsaturated fats and fiber.
- **Olive Oil:** Rich in monounsaturated fats and antioxidants.
- **Coconut Oil:** Contains medium-chain triglycerides (MCTs) that are easily digested and provide quick energy.

## 7. Herbs and Spices

Herbs and spices not only add flavor to your meals but also offer anti-inflammatory and antioxidant benefits:

- **Turmeric:** Contains curcumin, a powerful anti-inflammatory compound.
- **Ginger:** Helps reduce inflammation and soothe digestive issues.
- **Garlic:** Contains compounds that boost the immune system and reduce inflammation.
- **Cinnamon:** Helps regulate blood sugar levels and has anti-inflammatory properties.

# *FURTHER CLARIFIATION*

The inclusion of legumes and certain herbs and spices can indeed seem contradictory given their high FODMAP content. The reason for this apparent contradiction lies in individual variability and the nuanced approach needed for managing endometriosis with diet. Let me clarify:

**Understanding Individual Differences**

Not every person with endometriosis will have the same dietary triggers. While some individuals may find that high-FODMAP foods exacerbate their symptoms, others might tolerate them well and benefit from their nutritional value. Therefore, dietary recommendations need to be tailored to each person's unique sensitivities and nutritional needs.

**Legumes (Beans)**

Legumes like beans are excellent sources of plant-based protein, fiber, and essential nutrients. However, they are high in FODMAPs, which can cause digestive discomfort in some individuals. For those who tolerate them well, beans can be a valuable part of an anti-inflammatory diet. If you find that beans trigger your symptoms, you can opt for lower-FODMAP alternatives such as:

- **Lentils (in small amounts):** Particularly the canned variety, which tends to have lower FODMAP levels.
- **Firm Tofu:** A great plant-based protein source that is low in FODMAPs.

**Garlic**

Garlic is known for its anti-inflammatory and immune-boosting properties, making it beneficial for overall health. However, it is also high in FODMAPs. If you are sensitive to FODMAPs, you can still enjoy the flavor of garlic by using garlic-infused oils, which contain the flavor compounds without the FODMAP content.

**Tailoring Your Diet**

Here are some tips for tailoring your diet to manage endometriosis while considering FODMAP sensitivities:

1. **Elimination and Reintroduction:**
   - Start by eliminating high-FODMAP foods from your diet for a period (usually 6-8 weeks).
   - Gradually reintroduce these foods one at a time to identify which ones you can tolerate and which ones exacerbate your symptoms.
2. **Low-FODMAP Alternatives:**
   - Use low-FODMAP substitutes for high-FODMAP foods. For example, instead of garlic, use garlic-infused oil. Instead of beans, use lentils in small amounts or firm tofu.
3. **Portion Control:**
   - Sometimes, it's the quantity of FODMAPs that matters. Small amounts of high-FODMAP foods might be tolerated, even if larger amounts cause symptoms.

# Meal Planning Tips

## 1. Understand Your Nutritional Needs

Before you start meal planning, it's crucial to understand your nutritional needs. Endometriosis is an inflammatory condition, so your diet should focus on anti-inflammatory foods. Make sure to include a variety of fruits, vegetables, whole grains, lean proteins, and healthy fats. Consult with a nutritionist to create a personalized plan that meets your specific dietary requirements.

## 2. Incorporate Anti-Inflammatory Foods

Focus on foods that have anti-inflammatory properties. These include:

- **Fruits and Vegetables:** Aim for a rainbow of colors to ensure you're getting a wide range of nutrients and antioxidants. Berries, leafy greens, and cruciferous vegetables are particularly beneficial.
- **Omega-3 Fatty Acids:** Include fatty fish like salmon and mackerel, as well as plant-based sources like chia seeds, flaxseeds, and walnuts.
- **Whole Grains:** Opt for quinoa, brown rice, and oats, which provide fiber and essential nutrients without the inflammation associated with refined grains.
- **Herbs and Spices:** Use turmeric, ginger, garlic, and cinnamon to add flavor and anti-inflammatory benefits to your meals.

## 3. Avoid Trigger Foods

Identify and avoid foods that trigger your symptoms. Common culprits include:

- **Processed and Refined Foods:** These often contain unhealthy fats, sugars, and additives that can increase inflammation.
- **Sugary Foods and Beverages:** High sugar intake can lead to inflammation and insulin resistance, exacerbating endometriosis symptoms.
- **Dairy and Gluten:** Some women find relief by eliminating or reducing dairy and gluten. Experiment with alternatives to see if they make a difference for you.

## 4. Plan Balanced Meals

Ensure that each meal is balanced and includes a variety of nutrients. A balanced meal typically consists of:

- **Protein:** Lean meats, fish, beans, legumes, or plant-based proteins like tofu and tempeh.
- **Healthy Fats:** Avocados, nuts, seeds, and healthy oils like olive oil.
- **Complex Carbohydrates:** Whole grains and starchy vegetables like sweet potatoes and quinoa.
- **Fiber-Rich Vegetables:** Aim to fill half your plate with vegetables to boost nutrient intake and support digestive health.

### 5. Prep Ahead of Time

Preparing meals in advance can save time and reduce stress during busy days. Consider the following tips:

- **Batch Cooking:** Cook large quantities of staple foods like grains, beans, and roasted vegetables at the beginning of the week and use them in various meals.
- **Freezing Meals:** Prepare and freeze meals in individual portions for quick and easy access. Soups, stews, and casseroles freeze particularly well.
- **Prepping Ingredients:** Chop vegetables, marinate proteins, and prepare dressings or sauces in advance to streamline meal assembly.

### 6. Stay Organized

Keeping organized is key to successful meal planning. Use these strategies to stay on track:

- **Meal Planning Calendar:** Use a physical calendar or a digital app to plan your meals for the week. Note down breakfasts, lunches, dinners, and snacks.
- **Grocery Lists:** Create a detailed grocery list based on your meal plan to ensure you have all the ingredients you need and avoid impulse purchases.
- **Labeling and Storage:** Label prepped meals and ingredients with dates to keep track of freshness and ensure you use everything in a timely manner.

### 7. Incorporate Variety

Variety is essential to prevent meal fatigue and ensure a broad spectrum of nutrients. Rotate different types of fruits, vegetables, proteins, and grains in your meals. Experiment with new recipes and cooking methods to keep things interesting and enjoyable.

### 8. Listen to Your Body

Pay attention to how different foods affect your symptoms. Keep a food diary to track what you eat and how you feel afterward. This can help you identify patterns and make informed adjustments to your diet.

### 9. Stay Hydrated

Proper hydration is essential for overall health and can help manage endometriosis symptoms. Aim to drink at least eight glasses of water a day. Herbal teas, such as chamomile and ginger, can also be soothing and anti-inflammatory.

# *Grocery Shopping Guide*

**1. Plan Ahead**

Planning is key to a successful grocery shopping trip. Start by creating a meal plan for the week that includes breakfast, lunch, dinner, and snacks. Based on this plan, make a detailed shopping list. This will help you stay focused and avoid impulse purchases that may not align with your dietary needs.

**2. Shop the Perimeter**

Most grocery stores are set up so that fresh, whole foods are located around the perimeter. This includes produce, meats, dairy, and bakery sections. These areas tend to have less processed and more nutrient-dense options. Focus your shopping here to find the healthiest choices.

**3. Fruits and Vegetables**

Fruits and vegetables should make up a significant portion of your diet. They are rich in vitamins, minerals, and antioxidants that help combat inflammation. Aim for a variety of colors to ensure a wide range of nutrients:

- **Leafy Greens:** Spinach, kale, Swiss chard, and arugula.
- **Cruciferous Vegetables:** Broccoli, cauliflower, Brussels sprouts, and cabbage.
- **Berries:** Blueberries, strawberries, raspberries, and blackberries.
- **Citrus Fruits:** Oranges, lemons, limes, and grapefruits.
- **Other Vegetables:** Carrots, bell peppers, zucchini, and sweet potatoes.

**4. Whole Grains**

Whole grains provide fiber, which helps with digestion and maintaining stable blood sugar levels. Choose unrefined, whole grains such as:

- Quinoa
- Brown rice
- Oats
- Barley
- Millet

**5. Lean Proteins**

Protein is essential for muscle repair and overall health. Select lean sources of protein that are low in unhealthy fats:

- **Poultry:** Chicken and turkey.
- **Fish:** Salmon, mackerel, sardines, and trout (rich in omega-3 fatty acids).
- **Legumes:** Lentils, chickpeas, and black beans (opt for canned varieties labeled "no added salt" or prepare from dried to control sodium content).
- **Plant-Based Proteins:** Tofu, tempeh, and edamame.

## 6. Healthy Fats

Incorporating healthy fats into your diet helps reduce inflammation and supports hormone production:

- **Avocados**
- **Nuts and Seeds:** Almonds, walnuts, chia seeds, and flaxseeds.
- **Healthy Oils:** Olive oil, coconut oil, and avocado oil.

## 7. Dairy Alternatives

If you find that dairy exacerbates your symptoms, consider dairy alternatives:

- **Milk Alternatives:** Almond milk, coconut milk, and oat milk.
- **Cheese Alternatives:** Look for nut-based cheeses or those labeled as dairy-free.

## 8. Low-FODMAP Foods

If you are sensitive to FODMAPs, choose low-FODMAP foods to reduce digestive discomfort:

- **Low-FODMAP Fruits:** Bananas, blueberries, strawberries, and oranges.
- **Low-FODMAP Vegetables:** Carrots, zucchini, bell peppers, and spinach.
- **Other Low-FODMAP Items:** Firm tofu, tempeh, and certain gluten-free grains.

## 9. Herbs and Spices

Herbs and spices are essential for adding flavor and anti-inflammatory benefits to your meals:

- **Turmeric**
- **Ginger**
- **Garlic (use garlic-infused oil if sensitive to FODMAPs)**
- **Cinnamon**
- **Basil, oregano, thyme, and rosemary**

## 10. Reading Labels

Processed foods can hide unhealthy ingredients. Reading labels helps you make informed choices:

- **Check Ingredients:** Avoid foods with long lists of unrecognizable ingredients, artificial additives, and preservatives.
- **Watch for Added Sugars:** Look for natural sweeteners like honey or maple syrup, and avoid high-fructose corn syrup and other added sugars.
- **Monitor Sodium Content:** Choose products labeled "low sodium" or "no added salt" to avoid excessive sodium intake.

## 11. Shopping Local and Seasonal

Buying local and seasonal produce ensures you get the freshest, most nutrient-dense options. Farmers' markets are great places to find locally grown fruits and vegetables, and often, these foods are more flavorful and affordable.

**12. Consider Organic**
While not always necessary, choosing organic products can reduce your exposure to pesticides and other chemicals. Prioritize organic options for the "Dirty Dozen" – fruits and vegetables known to have higher pesticide residues.

**13. Stocking Your Pantry**
Keeping a well-stocked pantry makes meal preparation easier and ensures you always have healthy options on hand. Include:
- **Canned Beans and Lentils**
- **Whole Grains**
- **Nuts and Seeds**
- **Dried Herbs and Spices**
- **Healthy Oils**

# Breakfast Recipes

**1. Quinoa Porridge**

**Ingredients:**

- 1 cup quinoa, rinsed
- 2 cups almond milk (or any dairy-free milk)
- 1 cup water
- 1 tsp cinnamon
- 1 tsp vanilla extract
- 1 tbsp maple syrup (optional)
- 1/2 cup fresh berries (e.g., blueberries, strawberries)
- 2 tbsp chopped nuts (e.g., almonds, walnuts)

**Instructions:**

1. In a medium saucepan, combine the rinsed quinoa, almond milk, water, and cinnamon.
2. Bring to a boil over medium-high heat, then reduce to a simmer.
3. Cover and cook for 15 minutes, or until the quinoa is tender and the liquid is mostly absorbed.
4. Stir in the vanilla extract and maple syrup (if using).
5. Serve warm, topped with fresh berries and chopped nuts.

**Nutrition Info (per serving):**

- Calories: 220
- Protein: 6g
- Carbohydrates: 32g
- Fat: 8g
- Fiber: 4g
- Sugar: 6g

**Serves:**

4

**Cooking Time:**

20 minutes

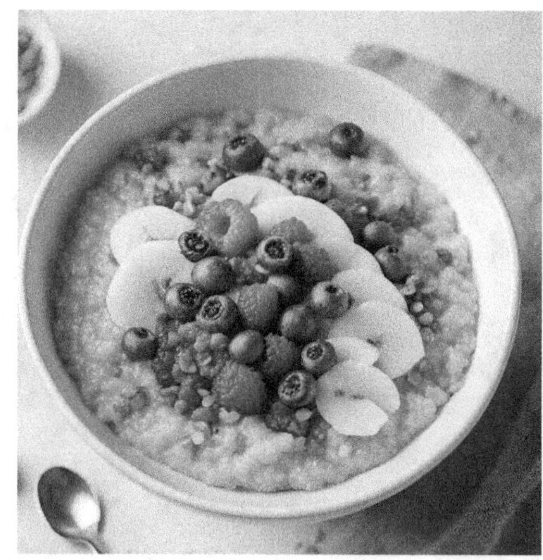

## 2. Chia Pudding

**Ingredients:**

- 1/4 cup chia seeds
- 1 cup coconut milk (or any dairy-free milk)
- 1 tbsp maple syrup or honey
- 1 tsp vanilla extract
- 1/2 cup fresh fruit (e.g., mango, berries)

**Instructions:**

1. In a bowl or mason jar, combine chia seeds, coconut milk, maple syrup, and vanilla extract.
2. Stir well to combine.
3. Cover and refrigerate for at least 4 hours, or overnight, until the mixture has thickened.
4. Stir the pudding to break up any clumps.
5. Serve topped with fresh fruit.

**Nutrition Info (per serving):**

- Calories: 190
- Protein: 4g
- Carbohydrates: 18g
- Fat: 12g
- Fiber: 10g
- Sugar: 8g

**Serves:**

2

**Cooking Time:**

10 minutes (plus 4 hours chilling time)

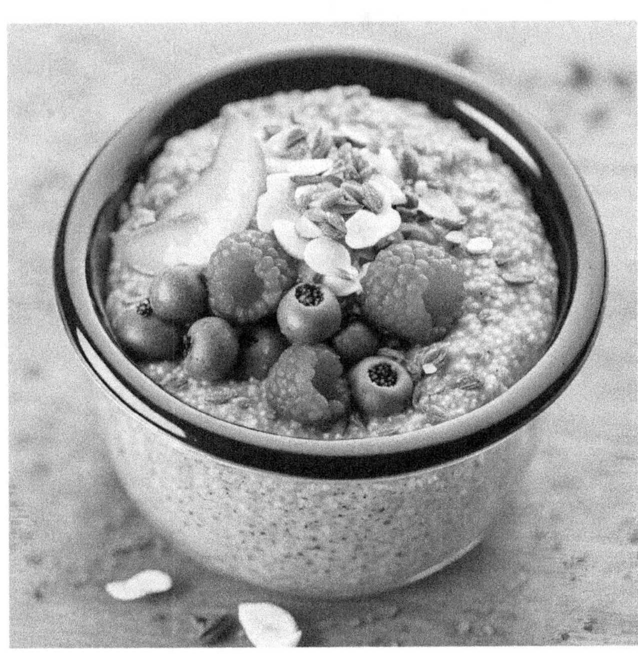

**3. Oatmeal with Flaxseeds**

**Ingredients:**

- 1 cup rolled oats
- 2 cups water or almond milk
- 1 tbsp ground flaxseeds
- 1/2 tsp cinnamon
- 1 banana, sliced
- 1 tbsp almond butter

**Instructions:**

1. In a medium saucepan, bring the water or almond milk to a boil.
2. Add the rolled oats and reduce heat to a simmer.
3. Cook for 5-7 minutes, stirring occasionally, until the oats are soft and creamy.
4. Stir in the ground flaxseeds and cinnamon.
5. Serve topped with sliced banana and a dollop of almond butter.

**Nutrition Info (per serving):**

- Calories: 250
- Protein: 7g
- Carbohydrates: 40g
- Fat: 9g
- Fiber: 8g
- Sugar: 8g

**Serves:**

2

**Cooking Time:**

10 minutes

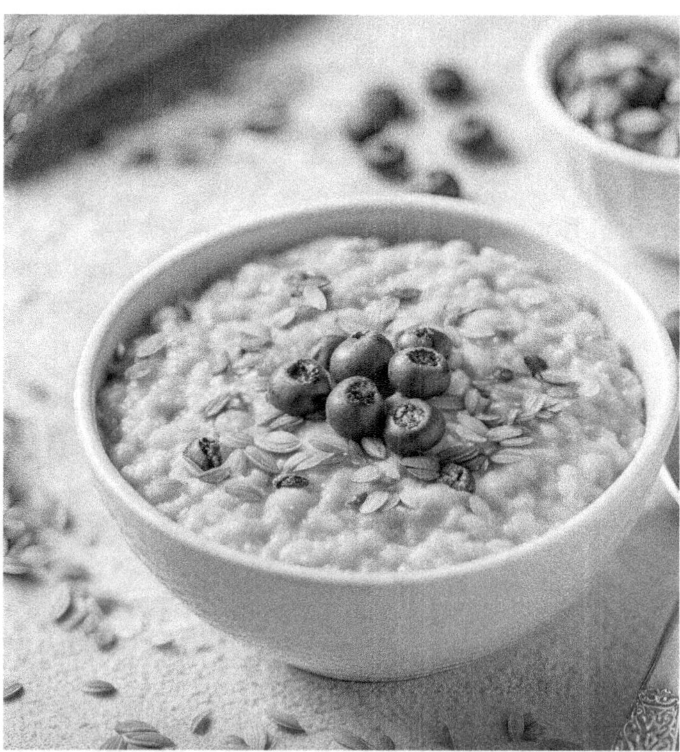

## 4. Buckwheat Pancakes

**Ingredients:**

- 1 cup buckwheat flour
- 1 tbsp coconut sugar or honey
- 1 tsp baking powder
- 1/2 tsp baking soda
- 1 cup almond milk (or any dairy-free milk)
- 1 tbsp apple cider vinegar
- 1 egg (or flax egg: 1 tbsp ground flaxseeds + 3 tbsp water)
- 1 tsp vanilla extract
- Coconut oil for cooking

**Instructions:**

1. In a medium bowl, mix the buckwheat flour, coconut sugar, baking powder, and baking soda.
2. In another bowl, whisk together the almond milk and apple cider vinegar. Let sit for a few minutes to curdle.
3. Add the egg and vanilla extract to the milk mixture, then pour into the dry ingredients.
4. Stir until just combined.
5. Heat a non-stick skillet over medium heat and lightly coat with coconut oil.
6. Pour 1/4 cup of batter onto the skillet for each pancake. Cook until bubbles form on the surface, then flip and cook until golden brown.
7. Serve warm with your favorite toppings like fresh berries or maple syrup.

**Nutrition Info (per serving):**

- Calories: 140
- Protein: 4g
- Carbohydrates: 24g
- Fat: 3g
- Fiber: 3g
- Sugar: 4g

**Serves:**

4

**Cooking Time:**

20 minutes

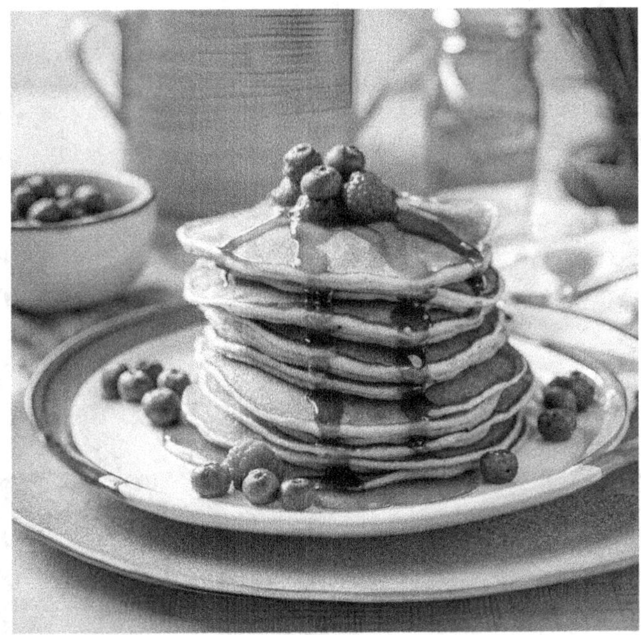

## 5. Turmeric Tofu Scramble

**Ingredients:**

- 1 block (14 oz) firm tofu, drained and crumbled
- 1 tbsp olive oil
- 1/2 tsp turmeric
- 1/2 tsp cumin
- 1/2 tsp paprika
- 1/4 tsp black pepper
- 1/2 red bell pepper, diced
- 1 small onion, diced
- 1 cup baby spinach
- 1 tbsp nutritional yeast (optional)

**Instructions:**

1. Heat the olive oil in a large skillet over medium heat.
2. Add the diced onion and red bell pepper. Sauté until softened, about 5 minutes.
3. Add the crumbled tofu, turmeric, cumin, paprika, and black pepper. Stir to combine and cook for another 5 minutes.
4. Stir in the baby spinach and cook until wilted, about 2 minutes.
5. Sprinkle with nutritional yeast, if using, and stir to combine.
6. Serve hot, with whole grain toast or as a filling for a breakfast burrito.

**Nutrition Info (per serving):**

- Calories: 200
- Protein: 14g
- Carbohydrates: 8g
- Fat: 14g
- Fiber: 3g
- Sugar: 2g

**Serves:**

4

**Cooking Time:**

15 minutes

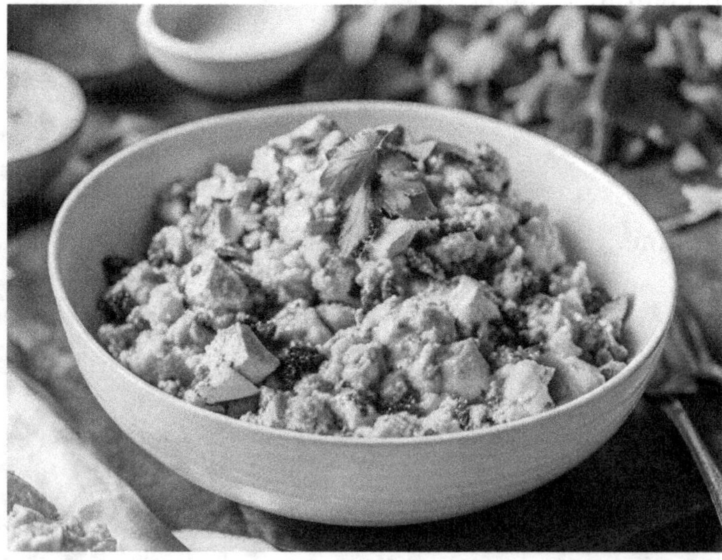

## 6. Almond Yogurt with Kiwi

**Ingredients:**

- 1 cup almond yogurt (unsweetened)
- 2 kiwis, peeled and sliced
- 1 tbsp chia seeds
- 1 tbsp honey or maple syrup (optional)
- 1 tbsp chopped almonds

**Instructions:**

1. Divide the almond yogurt into two bowls.
2. Top each bowl with sliced kiwis, chia seeds, and chopped almonds.
3. Drizzle with honey or maple syrup if desired.
4. Serve immediately.

**Nutrition Info (per serving):**

- Calories: 180
- Protein: 5g
- Carbohydrates: 25g
- Fat: 7g
- Fiber: 5g
- Sugar: 14g

**Serves:**

2

**Cooking Time:**

5 minutes

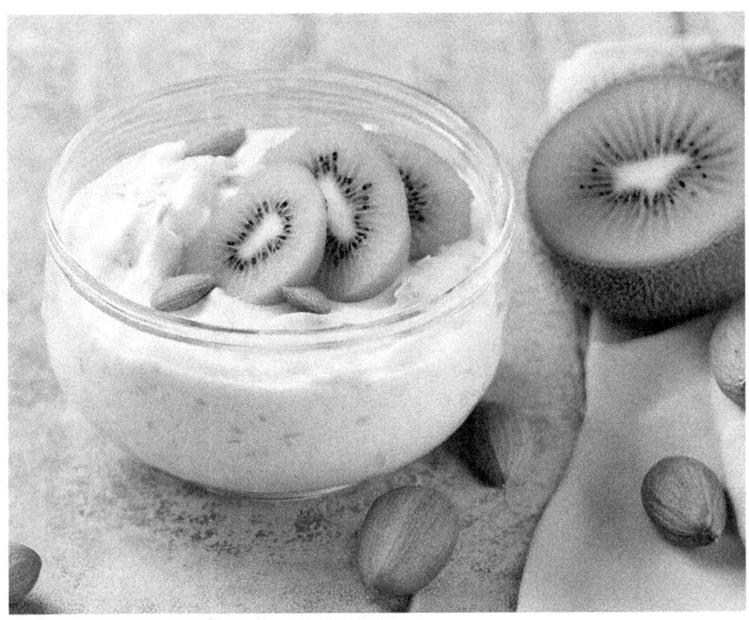

### 7. Banana Oat Cookies

**Ingredients:**

- 2 ripe bananas, mashed
- 1 cup rolled oats
- 1/4 cup almond butter
- 1/4 cup dark chocolate chips
- 1 tsp vanilla extract
- 1/2 tsp cinnamon

**Instructions:**

1. Preheat oven to 350°F (175°C) and line a baking sheet with parchment paper.
2. In a large bowl, mix the mashed bananas, rolled oats, almond butter, vanilla extract, and cinnamon until well combined.
3. Fold in the dark chocolate chips.
4. Drop spoonfuls of the mixture onto the prepared baking sheet and flatten slightly.
5. Bake for 15-20 minutes, or until the cookies are golden brown.
6. Let cool before serving.

**Nutrition Info (per serving, 2 cookies):**

- Calories: 150
- Protein: 4g
- Carbohydrates: 22g
- Fat: 6g
- Fiber: 4g
- Sugar: 8g

**Serves:**

12 cookies

**Cooking Time:**

25 minutes

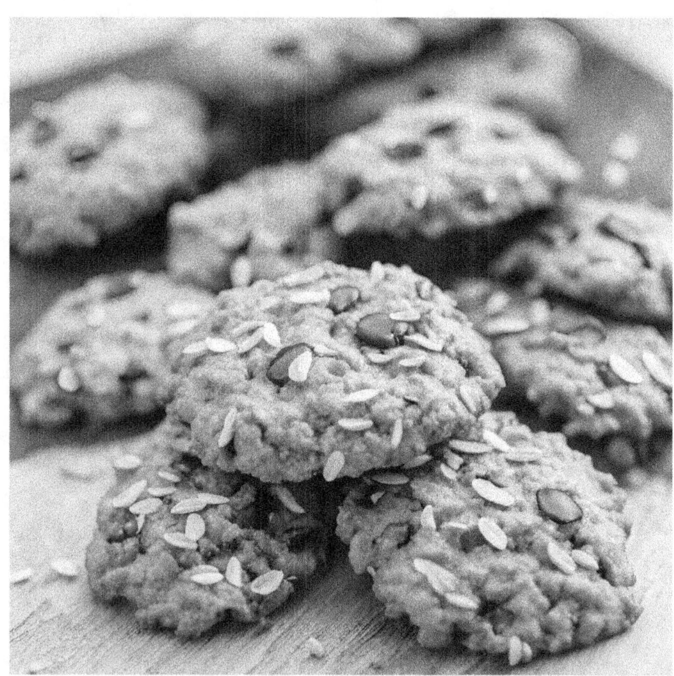

**8. Baked Avocado Eggs**

**Ingredients:**

- 2 ripe avocados, halved and pitted
- 4 large eggs
- 1/4 tsp paprika
- 1/4 tsp black pepper
- 1 tbsp chopped fresh chives

**Instructions:**

1. Preheat oven to 425°F (220°C).
2. Scoop out some of the avocado flesh to make enough room for the egg.
3. Place the avocado halves in a baking dish, ensuring they are stable.
4. Crack one egg into each avocado half.
5. Sprinkle with paprika and black pepper.
6. Bake for 15-20 minutes, or until the egg whites are set but the yolks are still slightly runny.
7. Sprinkle with fresh chives and serve immediately.

**Nutrition Info (per serving, 1 avocado half):**

- Calories: 240
- Protein: 9g
- Carbohydrates: 9g
- Fat: 21g
- Fiber: 7g
- Sugar: 1g

**Serves:**

4

**Cooking Time:**

20 minutes

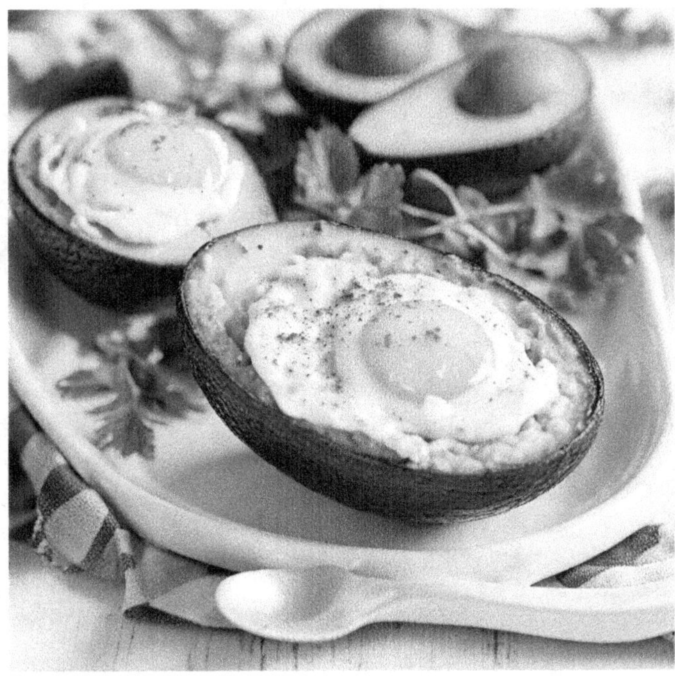

## 9. Berry and Coconut Smoothie

**Ingredients:**

- 1 cup mixed berries (fresh or frozen)
- 1 cup coconut milk (unsweetened)
- 1/2 banana
- 1 tbsp chia seeds
- 1 tsp vanilla extract

**Instructions:**

1. Combine all ingredients in a blender.
2. Blend until smooth and creamy.
3. Pour into glasses and serve immediately.

**Nutrition Info (per serving):**

- Calories: 180
- Protein: 2g
- Carbohydrates: 28g
- Fat: 8g
- Fiber: 7g
- Sugar: 14g

**Serves:**

2

**Cooking Time:**

5 minutes

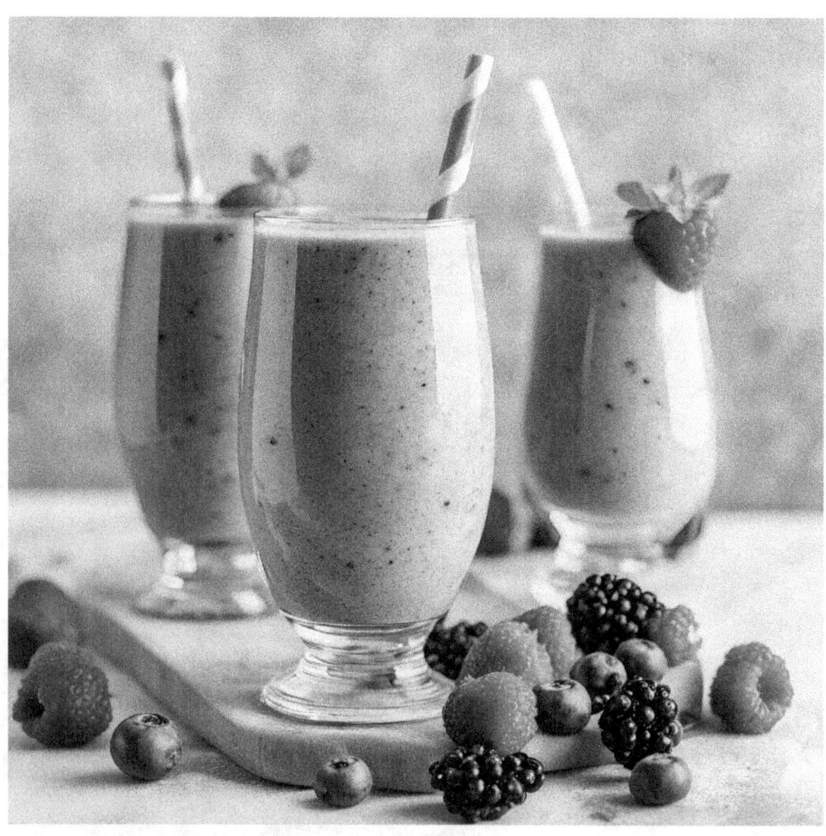

**10. Pumpkin Seed Granola**

**Ingredients:**

- 2 cups rolled oats
- 1/2 cup pumpkin seeds
- 1/4 cup chopped almonds
- 1/4 cup maple syrup or honey
- 1/4 cup coconut oil, melted
- 1 tsp vanilla extract
- 1/2 tsp cinnamon
- 1/2 cup dried cranberries (optional)

**Instructions:**

1. Preheat oven to 325°F (165°C) and line a baking sheet with parchment paper.
2. In a large bowl, combine the rolled oats, pumpkin seeds, and chopped almonds.
3. In a small bowl, whisk together the maple syrup, melted coconut oil, vanilla extract, and cinnamon.
4. Pour the wet ingredients over the dry ingredients and mix until well combined.
5. Spread the mixture evenly on the prepared baking sheet.
6. Bake for 20-25 minutes, stirring halfway through, until golden brown.
7. Let cool completely, then stir in the dried cranberries if using.
8. Store in an airtight container.

**Nutrition Info (per serving, 1/2 cup):**

- Calories: 250
- Protein: 6g
- Carbohydrates: 32g
- Fat: 12g
- Fiber: 4g
- Sugar: 10g

**Serves:**

8

**Cooking Time:**

30 minutes

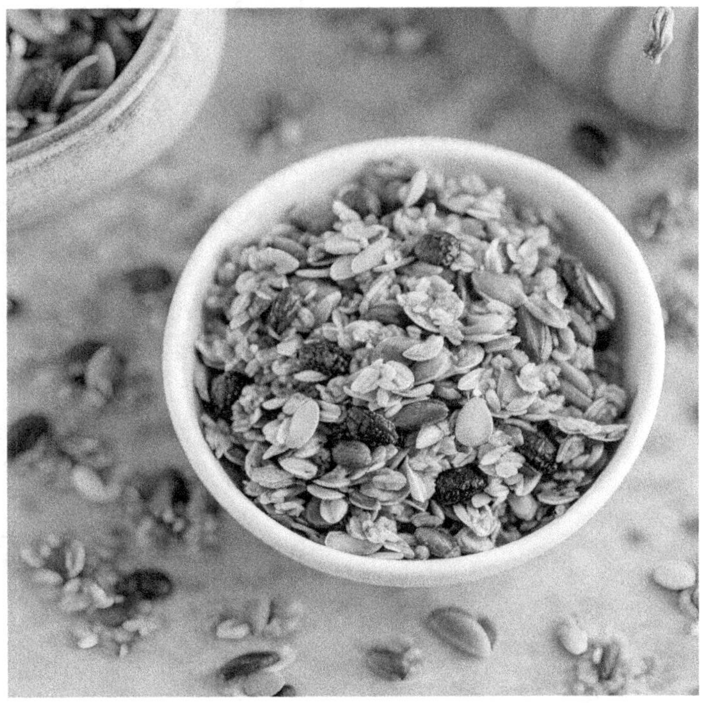

## 11. Spirulina Smoothie

**Ingredients:**

- 1 cup spinach
- 1 banana
- 1/2 cup pineapple chunks (fresh or frozen)
- 1 cup coconut water
- 1 tsp spirulina powder
- 1 tbsp chia seeds

**Instructions:**

1. Combine all ingredients in a blender.
2. Blend until smooth and creamy.
3. Pour into glasses and serve immediately.

**Nutrition Info (per serving):**

- Calories: 150
- Protein: 3g
- Carbohydrates: 32g
- Fat: 3g
- Fiber: 6g
- Sugar: 16g

**Serves:**

2

**Cooking Time:**

5 minutes

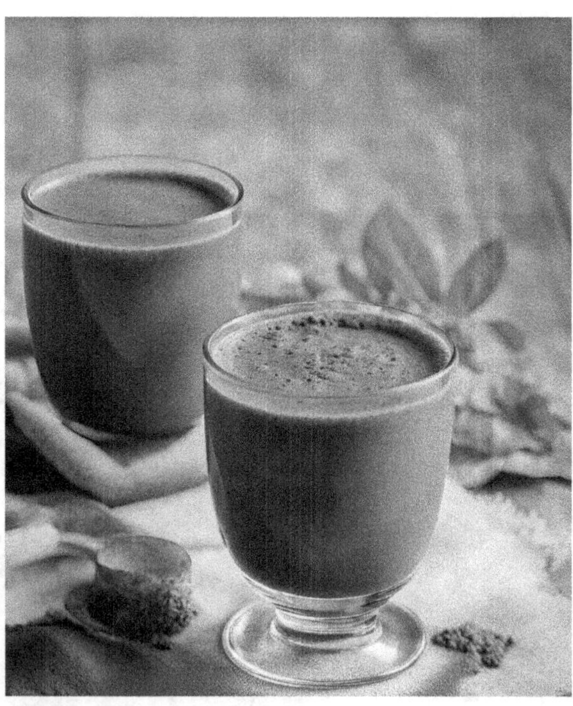

## 12. Millet Porridge

**Ingredients:**

- 1 cup millet, rinsed
- 3 cups water
- 1 cup almond milk (or any dairy-free milk)
- 1 tsp cinnamon
- 1 tbsp maple syrup (optional)
- 1/2 cup fresh berries (e.g., blueberries, raspberries)
- 2 tbsp chopped nuts (e.g., almonds, walnuts)

**Instructions:**

1. In a medium saucepan, combine the rinsed millet and water.
2. Bring to a boil, then reduce heat and simmer for about 20 minutes, or until the millet is tender.
3. Stir in the almond milk and cinnamon, cooking for another 5 minutes until the porridge thickens.
4. Sweeten with maple syrup if desired.
5. Serve topped with fresh berries and chopped nuts.

**Nutrition Info (per serving):**

- Calories: 210
- Protein: 6g
- Carbohydrates: 36g
- Fat: 5g
- Fiber: 4g
- Sugar: 6g

**Serves:**

4

**Cooking Time:**

30 minutes

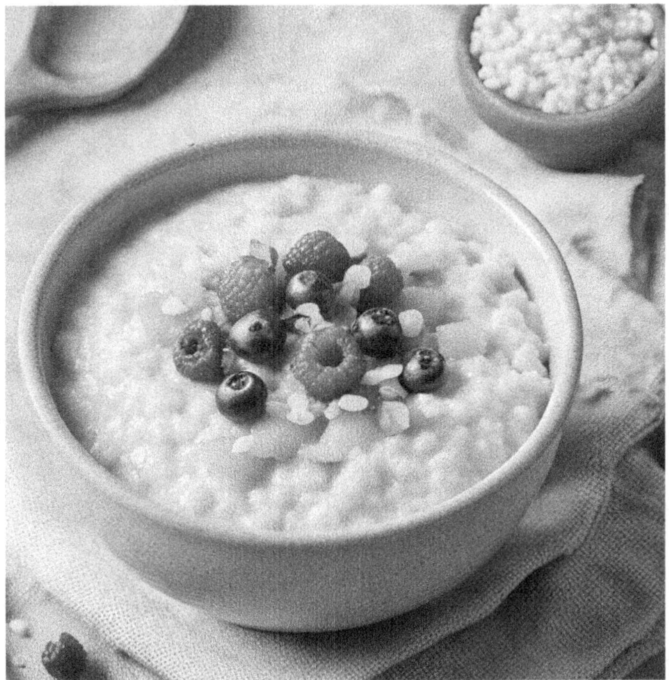

## 13. Rice Cakes with Almond Butter

**Ingredients:**

- 4 rice cakes
- 1/2 cup almond butter
- 1 banana, sliced
- 1 tbsp chia seeds
- 1 tbsp honey (optional)

**Instructions:**

1. Spread a layer of almond butter on each rice cake.
2. Top with banana slices and sprinkle with chia seeds.
3. Drizzle with honey if desired.
4. Serve immediately.

**Nutrition Info (per serving, 1 rice cake):**

- Calories: 150
- Protein: 4g
- Carbohydrates: 18g
- Fat: 8g
- Fiber: 3g
- Sugar: 6g

**Serves:**

4

**Cooking Time:**

5 minutes

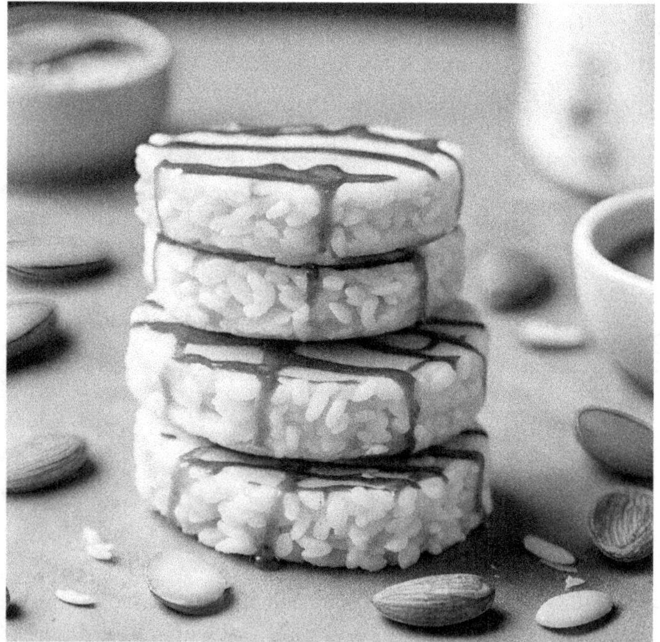

## 14. Stuffed Bell Peppers

**Ingredients:**
- 4 bell peppers, halved and seeds removed
- 1 cup cooked quinoa
- 1/2 cup black beans, rinsed and drained
- 1/2 cup corn kernels
- 1/2 cup diced tomatoes
- 1 tsp cumin
- 1/2 tsp paprika
- 1/4 tsp black pepper
- 1/4 cup chopped cilantro

**Instructions:**
1. Preheat oven to 375°F (190°C).
2. In a large bowl, combine the cooked quinoa, black beans, corn, diced tomatoes, cumin, paprika, and black pepper.
3. Stuff the bell pepper halves with the quinoa mixture.
4. Place the stuffed peppers in a baking dish and cover with foil.
5. Bake for 30-35 minutes, or until the peppers are tender.
6. Garnish with chopped cilantro and serve.

**Nutrition Info (per serving, 2 stuffed pepper halves):**
- Calories: 220
- Protein: 7g
- Carbohydrates: 38g
- Fat: 4g
- Fiber: 8g
- Sugar: 6g

**Serves:**

4

**Cooking Time:**

40 minutes

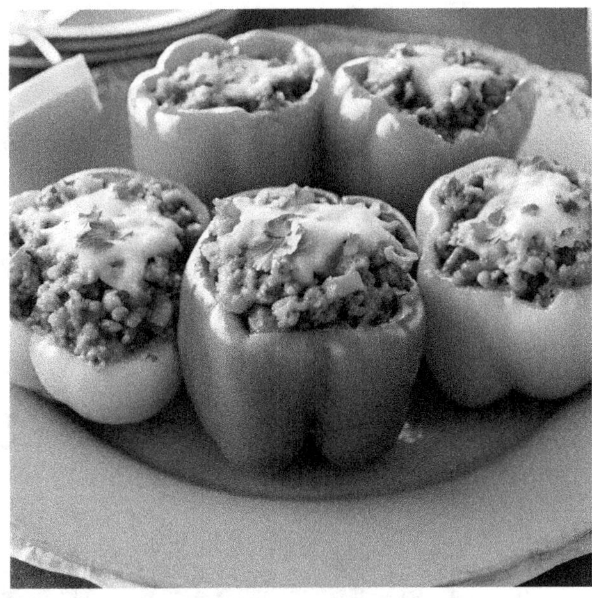

**15. Vegetable Omelette**

**Ingredients:**

- 4 large eggs
- 1/4 cup almond milk (or any dairy-free milk)
- 1/2 cup diced tomatoes
- 1/2 cup chopped spinach
- 1/4 cup diced onions
- 1/4 cup diced bell peppers
- 1 tbsp olive oil
- 1/4 tsp black pepper
- 1 tbsp chopped fresh herbs (e.g., parsley, chives)

**Instructions:**

1. In a bowl, whisk together the eggs, almond milk, and black pepper.
2. Heat the olive oil in a non-stick skillet over medium heat.
3. Add the onions and bell peppers, sautéing until softened.
4. Add the tomatoes and spinach, cooking until the spinach is wilted.
5. Pour the egg mixture over the vegetables.
6. Cook until the eggs are set, folding the omelette in half.
7. Garnish with fresh herbs and serve immediately.

**Nutrition Info (per serving):**

- Calories: 220
- Protein: 14g
- Carbohydrates: 6g
- Fat: 16g
- Fiber: 2g
- Sugar: 3g

**Serves:**

2

**Cooking Time:**

15 minutes

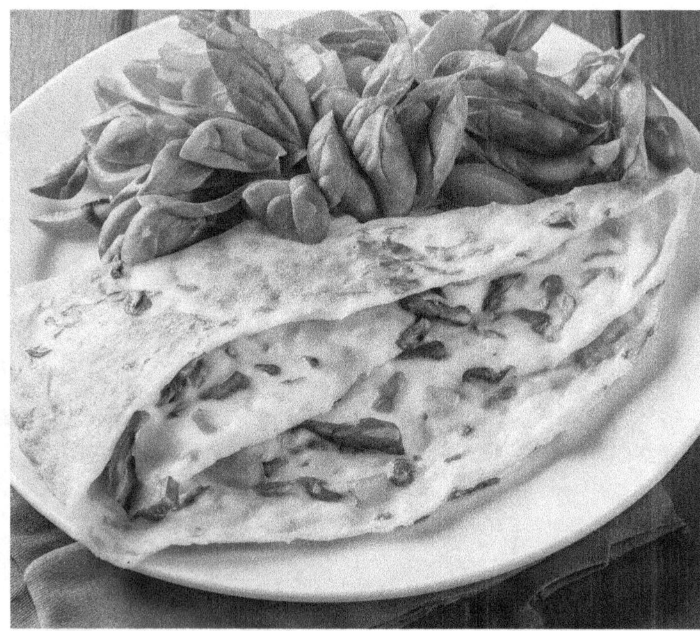

## 16. Zucchini Muffins

**Ingredients:**

- 1 1/2 cups grated zucchini
- 1 1/2 cups almond flour
- 1/2 cup rolled oats
- 1/4 cup honey or maple syrup
- 1/4 cup coconut oil, melted
- 2 large eggs
- 1 tsp vanilla extract
- 1 tsp cinnamon
- 1/2 tsp baking soda
- 1/2 tsp baking powder

**Instructions:**

1. Preheat oven to 350°F (175°C) and line a muffin tin with paper liners.
2. In a large bowl, combine the grated zucchini, almond flour, rolled oats, honey, coconut oil, eggs, vanilla extract, cinnamon, baking soda, and baking powder.
3. Mix until well combined.
4. Divide the batter evenly among the muffin cups.
5. Bake for 20-25 minutes, or until a toothpick inserted into the center comes out clean.
6. Let cool before serving.

**Nutrition Info (per serving, 1 muffin):**

- Calories: 150
- Protein: 4g
- Carbohydrates: 12g
- Fat: 10g
- Fiber: 3g
- Sugar: 7g

**Serves:**

12 muffins

**Cooking Time:**

30 minutes

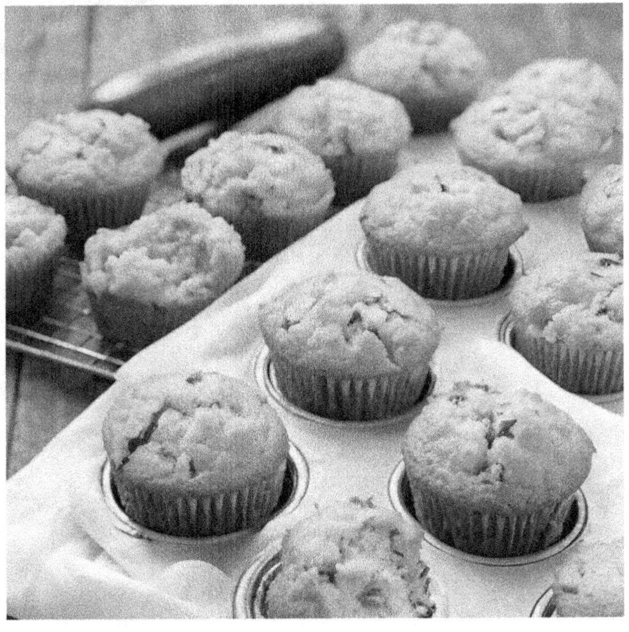

**17. Fruit Salad**

**Ingredients:**

- 1 cup strawberries, hulled and sliced
- 1 cup blueberries
- 1 cup pineapple chunks
- 1 kiwi, peeled and sliced
- 1 orange, peeled and segmented
- 1 tbsp fresh mint leaves, chopped
- 1 tbsp lime juice

**Instructions:**

1. In a large bowl, combine the strawberries, blueberries, pineapple chunks, kiwi, and orange segments.
2. Sprinkle with chopped mint leaves and drizzle with lime juice.
3. Toss gently to combine.
4. Serve immediately or chill for later.

**Nutrition Info (per serving):**

- Calories: 70
- Protein: 1g
- Carbohydrates: 17g
- Fat: 0g
- Fiber: 3g
- Sugar: 13g

**Serves:**

4

**Cooking Time:**

10 minutes

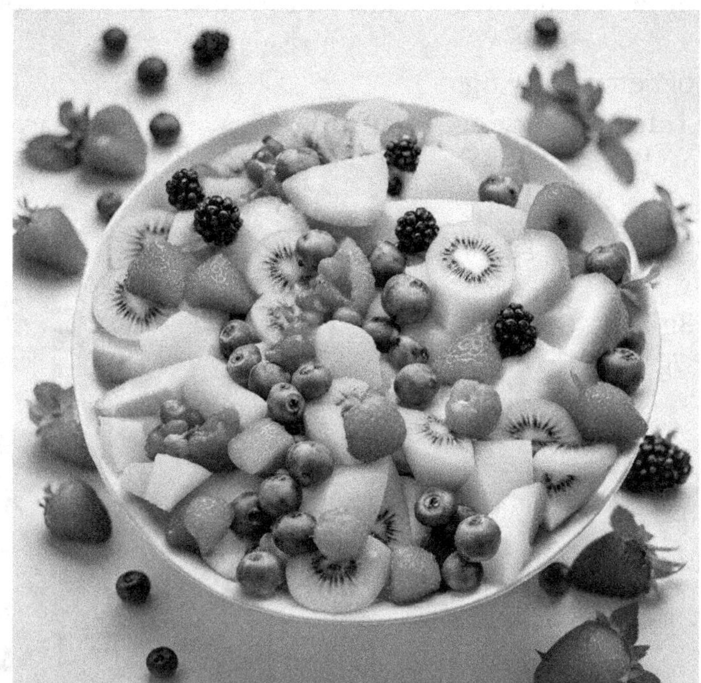

## 18. Sautéed Kale and Mushrooms

**Ingredients:**

- 1 bunch kale, washed and chopped
- 1 cup mushrooms, sliced
- 1 tbsp olive oil
- 1 garlic clove, minced
- 1/4 tsp red pepper flakes (optional)
- 1 tbsp lemon juice

**Instructions:**

1. Heat olive oil in a large skillet over medium heat.
2. Add the garlic and red pepper flakes (if using) and sauté for 1-2 minutes until fragrant.
3. Add the mushrooms and cook for about 5 minutes until they start to brown.
4. Add the kale and cook for another 5 minutes, stirring frequently, until wilted.
5. Drizzle with lemon juice and serve immediately.

**Nutrition Info (per serving):**

- Calories: 120
- Protein: 4g
- Carbohydrates: 12g
- Fat: 7g
- Fiber: 3g
- Sugar: 2g

**Serves:**

2

**Cooking Time:**

15 minutes

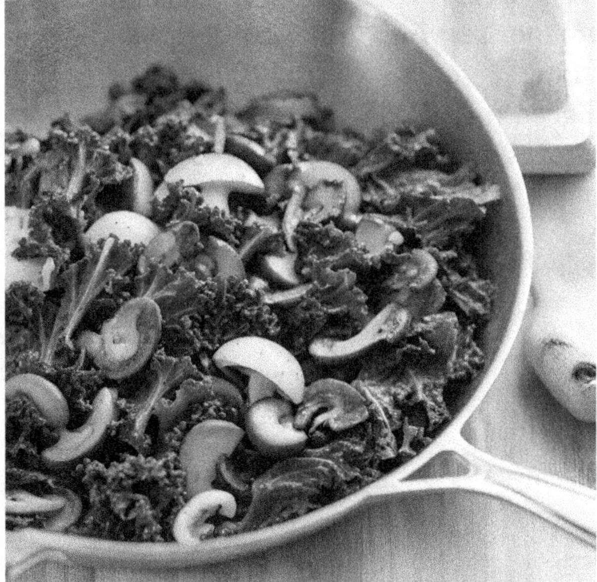

## 19. Raspberry Almond Muffins

**Ingredients:**

- 1 1/2 cups almond flour
- 1/2 cup rolled oats
- 1/2 cup raspberries (fresh or frozen)
- 1/4 cup honey or maple syrup
- 1/4 cup coconut oil, melted
- 2 large eggs
- 1 tsp vanilla extract
- 1 tsp baking powder
- 1/2 tsp baking soda

**Instructions:**

1. Preheat oven to 350°F (175°C) and line a muffin tin with paper liners.
2. In a large bowl, mix almond flour, rolled oats, baking powder, and baking soda.
3. In another bowl, whisk together the eggs, honey, coconut oil, and vanilla extract.
4. Combine the wet and dry ingredients, then gently fold in the raspberries.
5. Divide the batter evenly among the muffin cups.
6. Bake for 20-25 minutes, or until a toothpick inserted into the center comes out clean.
7. Let cool before serving.

**Nutrition Info (per serving, 1 muffin):**

- Calories: 160
- Protein: 5g
- Carbohydrates: 15g
- Fat: 10g
- Fiber: 3g
- Sugar: 7g

**Serves:**

12 muffins

**Cooking Time:**

30 minutes

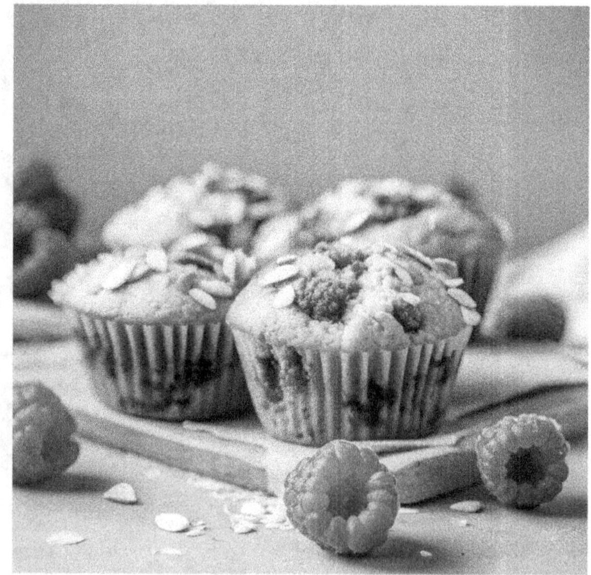

## 20. Pineapple and Cucumber Salad

**Ingredients:**

- 2 cups pineapple chunks
- 1 cucumber, sliced
- 1/4 cup red onion, thinly sliced
- 1 tbsp lime juice
- 1 tbsp chopped fresh mint

**Instructions:**

1. In a large bowl, combine the pineapple chunks, cucumber slices, and red onion.
2. Drizzle with lime juice and toss gently.
3. Sprinkle with chopped fresh mint.
4. Serve immediately or chill for later.

**Nutrition Info (per serving):**

- Calories: 60
- Protein: 1g
- Carbohydrates: 15g
- Fat: 0g
- Fiber: 2g
- Sugar: 12g

**Serves:**

4

**Cooking Time:**

10 minutes

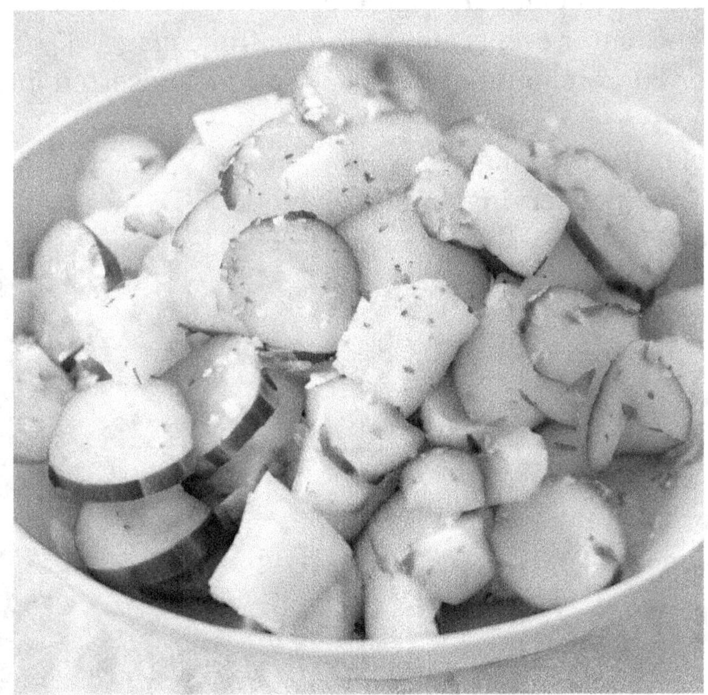

## 21. Sweet Potato Muffins

**Ingredients:**

- 1 cup mashed sweet potatoes (about 1 large sweet potato, cooked and mashed)
- 1 cup almond flour
- 1/2 cup rolled oats
- 1/4 cup honey or maple syrup
- 1/4 cup coconut oil, melted
- 2 large eggs
- 1 tsp vanilla extract
- 1 tsp cinnamon
- 1/2 tsp baking soda
- 1/2 tsp baking powder

**Instructions:**

1. Preheat oven to 350°F (175°C) and line a muffin tin with paper liners.
2. In a large bowl, mix almond flour, rolled oats, cinnamon, baking soda, and baking powder.
3. In another bowl, whisk together the mashed sweet potatoes, eggs, honey, coconut oil, and vanilla extract.
4. Combine the wet and dry ingredients until well mixed.
5. Divide the batter evenly among the muffin cups.
6. Bake for 20-25 minutes, or until a toothpick inserted into the center comes out clean.
7. Let cool before serving.

**Nutrition Info (per serving, 1 muffin):**

- Calories: 170
- Protein: 4g
- Carbohydrates: 22g
- Fat: 8g
- Fiber: 3g
- Sugar: 9g

**Serves:**

12 muffins

**Cooking Time:**

30 minutes

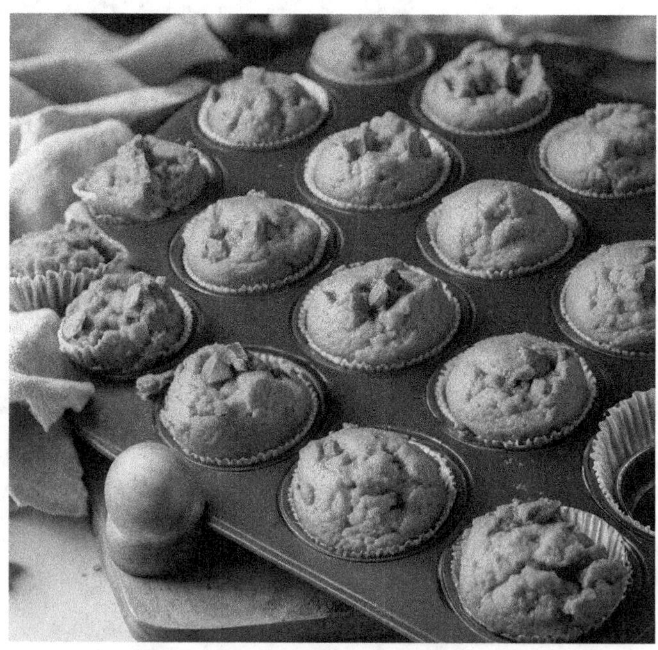

## 22. Spinach and Mushroom Crepes

**Ingredients:**

**For the crepes:**
- 1 cup chickpea flour
- 1 1/4 cups water
- 1 tbsp olive oil
- 1/2 tsp cumin

**For the filling:**
- 1 cup mushrooms, sliced
- 1 cup spinach, chopped
- 1 tbsp olive oil
- 1 garlic clove, minced
- 1/4 tsp black pepper

**Instructions:**

1. In a bowl, whisk together the chickpea flour, water, olive oil, and cumin until smooth. Let the batter rest for 15 minutes.
2. Heat a non-stick skillet over medium heat and lightly grease with olive oil.
3. Pour 1/4 cup of batter into the skillet, tilting to spread evenly. Cook until edges start to lift, then flip and cook the other side. Repeat with remaining batter.
4. For the filling, heat 1 tbsp olive oil in a skillet over medium heat. Add garlic and mushrooms, cooking until mushrooms are soft. Add spinach and cook until wilted.
5. Fill each crepe with the mushroom and spinach mixture.
6. Serve immediately.

**Nutrition Info (per serving, 2 crepes):**
- Calories: 220
- Protein: 8g
- Carbohydrates: 30g
- Fat: 8g
- Fiber: 5g
- Sugar: 3g

**Serves:**

4

**Cooking Time:**

30 minutes

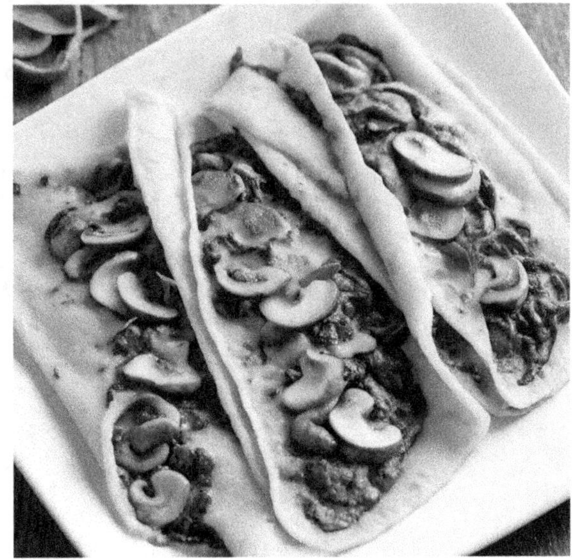

## 23. Walnut and Banana Pancakes

**Ingredients:**

- 1 cup rolled oats
- 1/2 cup walnuts, finely chopped
- 2 ripe bananas, mashed
- 1 cup almond milk (or any dairy-free milk)
- 1 tsp baking powder
- 1/2 tsp cinnamon
- 1 tsp vanilla extract
- Coconut oil for cooking

**Instructions:**

1. In a blender, blend the rolled oats until they form a flour-like consistency.
2. In a bowl, mix the oat flour, walnuts, baking powder, and cinnamon.
3. In another bowl, combine the mashed bananas, almond milk, and vanilla extract.
4. Pour the wet ingredients into the dry ingredients and mix until combined.
5. Heat a non-stick skillet over medium heat and lightly coat with coconut oil.
6. Pour 1/4 cup of batter onto the skillet for each pancake. Cook until bubbles form on the surface, then flip and cook until golden brown.
7. Serve warm with your favorite toppings.

**Nutrition Info (per serving):**

- Calories: 200
- Protein: 5g
- Carbohydrates: 28g
- Fat: 8g
- Fiber: 4g
- Sugar: 9g

**Serves:**

4

**Cooking Time:**

20 minutes

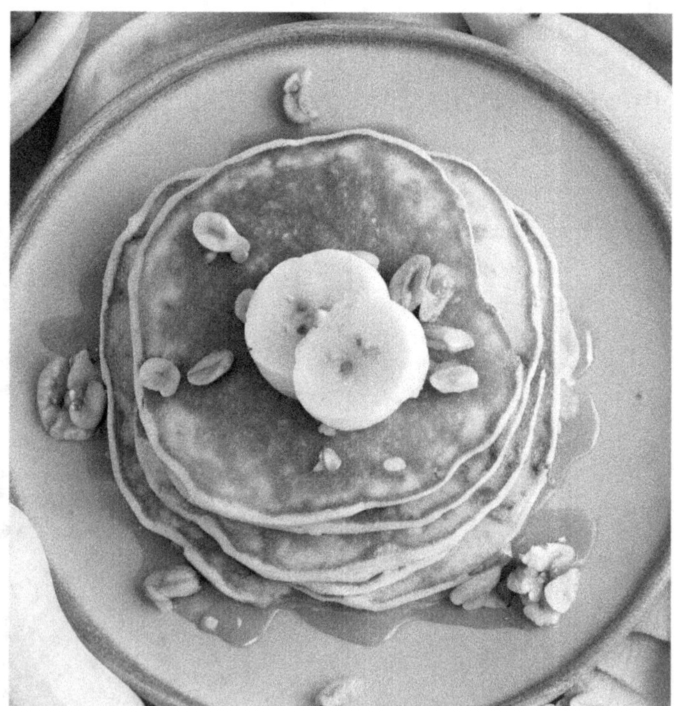

**24. Homemade Seed Bread**

**Ingredients:**
- 1 cup sunflower seeds
- 1/2 cup pumpkin seeds
- 1/2 cup chia seeds
- 1/2 cup ground flaxseeds
- 2 cups rolled oats
- 1/4 cup psyllium husk powder
- 1/4 cup coconut oil, melted
- 1 1/2 cups water
- 1 tbsp maple syrup

**Instructions:**
1. Preheat oven to 350°F (175°C) and line a loaf pan with parchment paper.
2. In a large bowl, combine the sunflower seeds, pumpkin seeds, chia seeds, ground flaxseeds, rolled oats, and psyllium husk powder.
3. In another bowl, whisk together the melted coconut oil, water, and maple syrup.
4. Pour the wet ingredients into the dry ingredients and mix until well combined. Let the mixture sit for at least 2 hours, or overnight.
5. Pour the mixture into the prepared loaf pan and smooth the top.
6. Bake for 50-60 minutes, or until the bread is firm and golden brown.
7. Let cool before slicing.

**Nutrition Info (per serving, 1 slice):**
- Calories: 200
- Protein: 6g
- Carbohydrates: 15g
- Fat: 12g
- Fiber: 6g
- Sugar: 2g

**Serves:**
10 slices

**Cooking Time:**
60 minutes

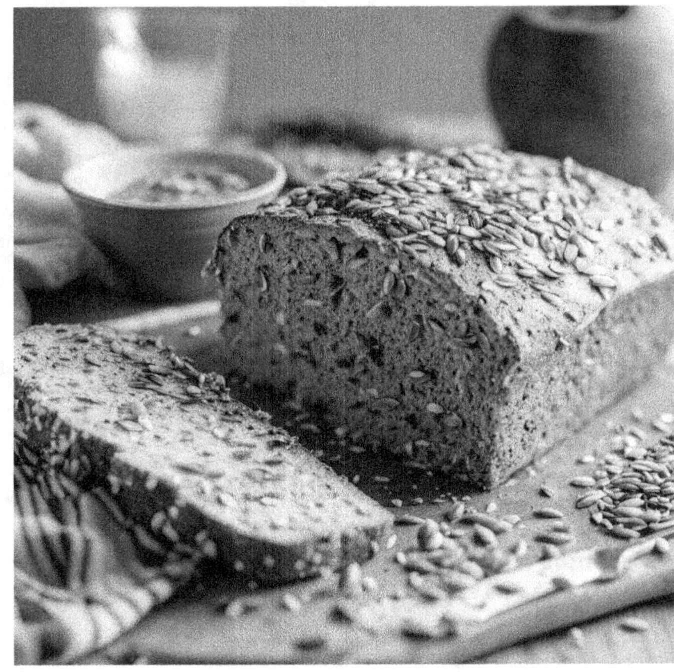

## 25. Grilled Asparagus and Tomato Skewers

**Ingredients:**

- 1 bunch asparagus, trimmed and cut into 2-inch pieces
- 1 pint cherry tomatoes
- 2 tbsp olive oil
- 1 tsp balsamic vinegar
- 1/4 tsp black pepper
- 1 tbsp fresh basil, chopped

**Instructions:**

1. Preheat grill to medium heat.
2. In a bowl, toss the asparagus and cherry tomatoes with olive oil and black pepper.
3. Thread the asparagus and tomatoes onto skewers.
4. Grill for 8-10 minutes, turning occasionally, until vegetables are tender and slightly charred.
5. Drizzle with balsamic vinegar and sprinkle with fresh basil before serving.

**Nutrition Info (per serving, 2 skewers):**

- Calories: 90
- Protein: 2g
- Carbohydrates: 8g
- Fat: 6g
- Fiber: 3g
- Sugar: 4g

**Serves:**

4

**Cooking Time:**

15 minutes

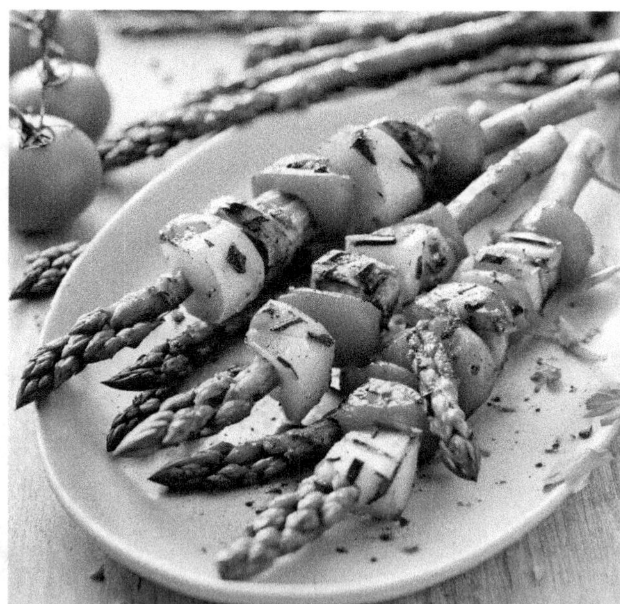

# Fish and Seafood

## 1. Peppered Mackerel with Salad

**Ingredients:**

- 4 mackerel fillets
- 2 tbsp olive oil
- 1 tsp ground black pepper
- 1 garlic clove, minced
- 1 lemon, sliced
- Mixed greens (e.g., arugula, spinach, lettuce)
- 1 cucumber, sliced
- 1 cup cherry tomatoes, halved
- 1/4 cup red onion, thinly sliced
- 2 tbsp balsamic vinaigrette

**Instructions:**

1. Preheat oven to 375°F (190°C).
2. Place the mackerel fillets on a baking sheet lined with parchment paper.
3. In a small bowl, mix olive oil, ground black pepper, and minced garlic.
4. Brush the mackerel fillets with the olive oil mixture and place lemon slices on top.
5. Bake for 15-20 minutes, or until the fish is cooked through and flakes easily with a fork.
6. While the fish is baking, prepare the salad by tossing mixed greens, cucumber, cherry tomatoes, and red onion in a bowl.
7. Drizzle the salad with balsamic vinaigrette and toss to combine.
8. Serve the baked mackerel with the salad.

**Nutrition Info (per serving):**

- Calories: 350
- Protein: 26g
- Carbohydrates: 10g
- Fat: 24g
- Fiber: 3g
- Sugar: 4g

**Serves:**

4

**Cooking Time:**

25 minutes

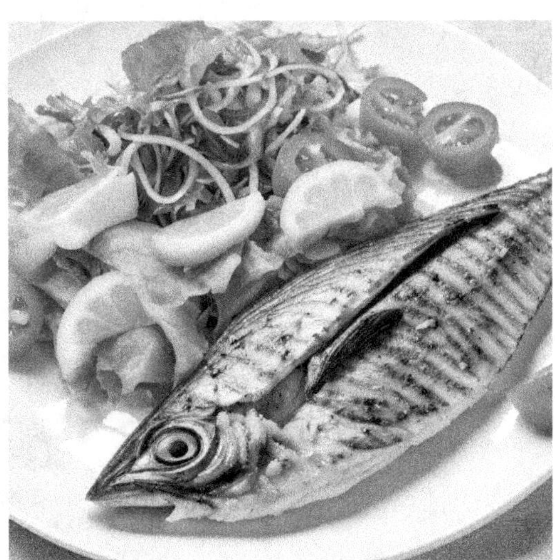

## 2. Shrimp and Spinach Frittata

**Ingredients:**

- 1/2 lb shrimp, peeled and deveined
- 1 tbsp olive oil
- 1 garlic clove, minced
- 1 cup baby spinach
- 6 large eggs
- 1/4 cup almond milk (or any dairy-free milk)
- 1/4 tsp black pepper
- 1 tbsp fresh dill, chopped

**Instructions:**

1. Preheat oven to 350°F (175°C).
2. Heat olive oil in a large oven-safe skillet over medium heat.
3. Add the minced garlic and cook for 1-2 minutes until fragrant.
4. Add the shrimp and cook until they turn pink, about 3-4 minutes.
5. Add the baby spinach and cook until wilted, about 2 minutes.
6. In a bowl, whisk together the eggs, almond milk, and black pepper.
7. Pour the egg mixture over the shrimp and spinach in the skillet.
8. Cook on the stovetop for 2-3 minutes until the edges start to set.
9. Transfer the skillet to the oven and bake for 10-15 minutes, or until the frittata is set and golden brown.
10. Garnish with fresh dill and serve.

**Nutrition Info (per serving):**

- Calories: 220
- Protein: 20g
- Carbohydrates: 3g
- Fat: 14g
- Fiber: 1g
- Sugar: 1g

**Serves:**

4

**Cooking Time:**

25 minutes

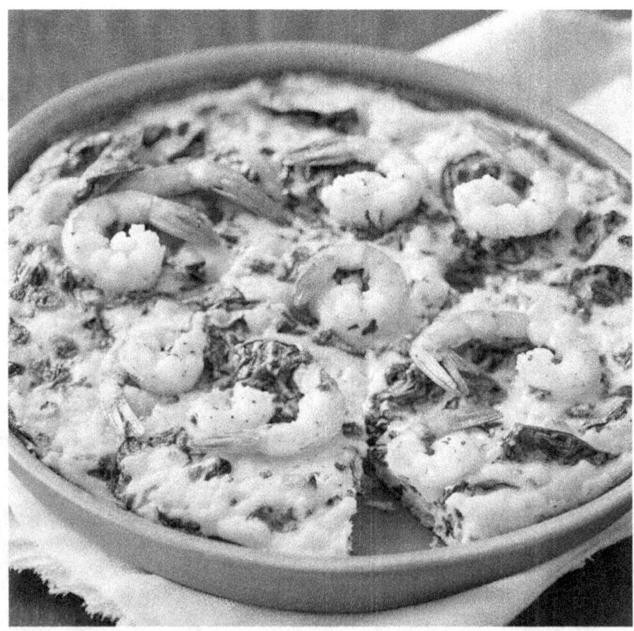

## 3. Perch with Roasted Almond Slivers

**Ingredients:**

- 4 perch fillets
- 2 tbsp olive oil
- 1/4 cup almond slivers
- 1 lemon, juiced
- 1 garlic clove, minced
- 1 tbsp fresh parsley, chopped

**Instructions:**

1. Preheat oven to 375°F (190°C).
2. Place the perch fillets on a baking sheet lined with parchment paper.
3. In a small bowl, mix olive oil, lemon juice, and minced garlic.
4. Brush the perch fillets with the olive oil mixture.
5. Sprinkle the almond slivers over the fillets.
6. Bake for 15-20 minutes, or until the fish is cooked through and flakes easily with a fork.
7. Garnish with fresh parsley and serve immediately.

**Nutrition Info (per serving):**

- Calories: 280
- Protein: 24g
- Carbohydrates: 2g
- Fat: 20g
- Fiber: 1g
- Sugar: 1g

**Serves:**

4

**Cooking Time:**

20 minutes

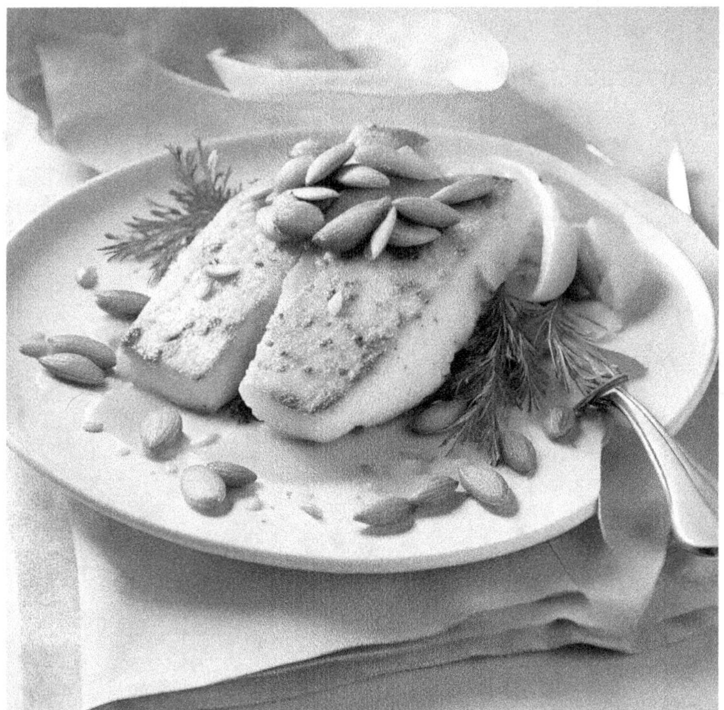

**4. Tilapia Piccata without Capers**

**Ingredients:**

- 4 tilapia fillets
- 2 tbsp olive oil
- 1/2 cup chicken broth (low sodium)
- 1/4 cup lemon juice
- 2 tbsp almond flour
- 1 garlic clove, minced
- 1 tbsp fresh parsley, chopped

**Instructions:**

1. Heat olive oil in a large skillet over medium-high heat.
2. Dredge the tilapia fillets in almond flour, shaking off excess.
3. Cook the tilapia in the skillet until golden brown and cooked through, about 3-4 minutes per side.
4. Remove the fish from the skillet and set aside.
5. In the same skillet, add the minced garlic and cook for 1 minute until fragrant.
6. Add the chicken broth and lemon juice, stirring to combine.
7. Bring to a simmer and cook for 2-3 minutes until slightly reduced.
8. Return the tilapia to the skillet and spoon the sauce over the fillets.
9. Garnish with fresh parsley and serve.

**Nutrition Info (per serving):**

- Calories: 240
- Protein: 25g
- Carbohydrates: 3g
- Fat: 14g
- Fiber: 1g
- Sugar: 1g

**Serves:**

4

**Cooking Time:**

20 minutes

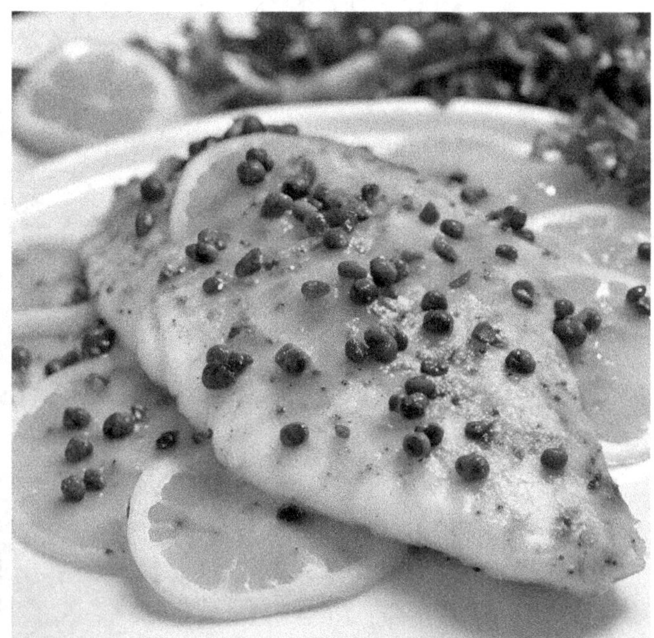

# 5. Kingfish Sashimi with Soy and Wasabi

**Ingredients:**

- 1 lb kingfish fillet, thinly sliced
- 1/4 cup low-sodium soy sauce
- 1 tbsp wasabi paste
- 1 lemon, thinly sliced
- 1 tbsp pickled ginger
- 1 tbsp sesame seeds
- 2 tbsp fresh chives, finely chopped

**Instructions:**

1. Arrange the thinly sliced kingfish on a serving platter.
2. In a small bowl, mix the soy sauce and wasabi paste until well combined.
3. Garnish the sashimi with lemon slices, pickled ginger, sesame seeds, and fresh chives.
4. Serve immediately with the soy and wasabi mixture on the side.

**Nutrition Info (per serving):**

- Calories: 150
- Protein: 26g
- Carbohydrates: 3g
- Fat: 4g
- Fiber: 1g
- Sugar: 1g

**Serves:**

4

**Cooking Time:**

10 minutes

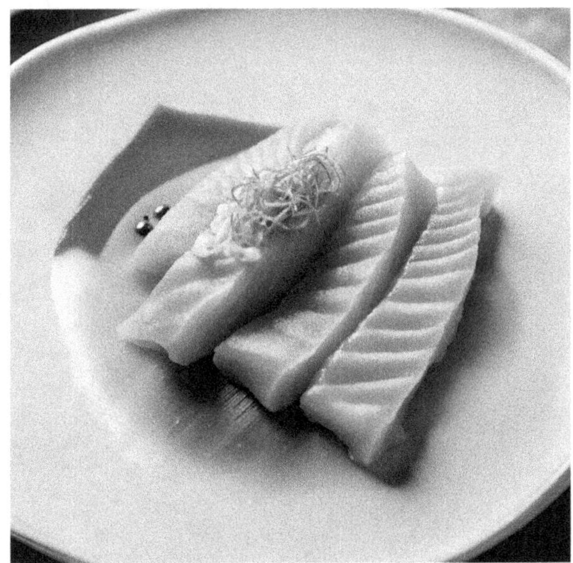

**6. Crab Stuffed Mushrooms**
**Ingredients:**

- 12 large mushroom caps
- 1 cup crab meat, drained and flaked
- 1/4 cup almond flour
- 2 tbsp olive oil
- 1 garlic clove, minced
- 1/4 tsp paprika
- 1 tbsp lemon juice
- 1 tbsp fresh parsley, chopped

**Instructions:**

1. Preheat oven to 375°F (190°C).
2. Remove the stems from the mushroom caps and set aside.
3. In a bowl, mix the crab meat, almond flour, olive oil, minced garlic, paprika, lemon juice, and chopped parsley.
4. Fill each mushroom cap with the crab mixture and place them on a baking sheet.
5. Bake for 15-20 minutes, or until the mushrooms are tender and the filling is golden brown.
6. Serve warm.

**Nutrition Info (per serving, 3 mushrooms):**

- Calories: 120
- Protein: 10g
- Carbohydrates: 5g
- Fat: 7g
- Fiber: 2g
- Sugar: 1g

**Serves:**

4

**Cooking Time:**

25 minutes

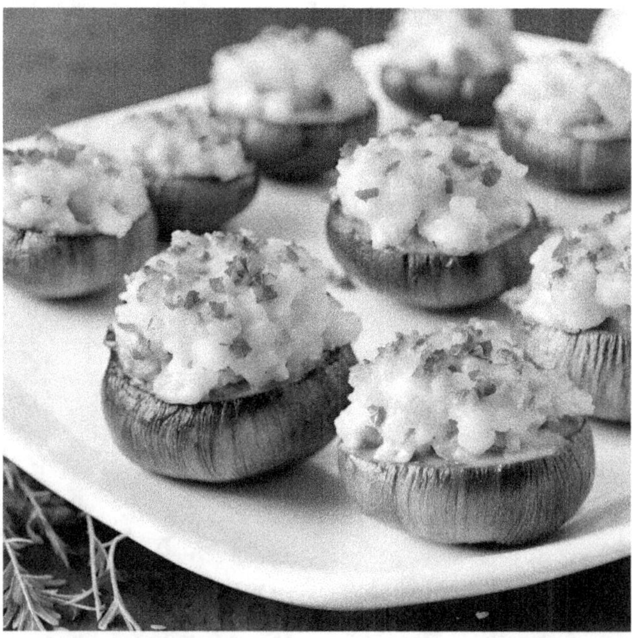

## 7. Lemon Butter Barramundi

**Ingredients:**

- 4 barramundi fillets
- 3 tbsp olive oil
- 2 tbsp lemon juice
- 2 tbsp fresh parsley, chopped
- 2 garlic cloves, minced
- 1/4 tsp black pepper
- Lemon slices for garnish

**Instructions:**

1. Preheat oven to 400°F (200°C).
2. In a small bowl, mix the olive oil, lemon juice, parsley, minced garlic, and black pepper.
3. Place the barramundi fillets on a baking sheet lined with parchment paper.
4. Brush the fillets with the lemon butter mixture.
5. Bake for 12-15 minutes, or until the fish is opaque and flakes easily with a fork.
6. Garnish with lemon slices and serve immediately.

**Nutrition Info (per serving):**

- Calories: 220
- Protein: 25g
- Carbohydrates: 2g
- Fat: 13g
- Fiber: 1g
- Sugar: 0g

**Serves:**

4

**Cooking Time:**

20 minutes

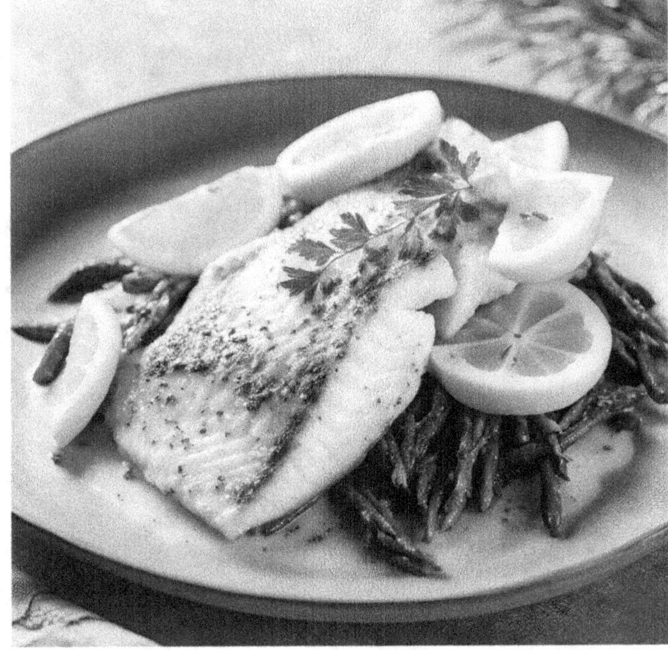

## 8. Pescado Zarandeado (Grilled Snapper)

**Ingredients:**

- 1 whole snapper, cleaned and scaled
- 1/4 cup olive oil
- 1/4 cup lime juice
- 2 garlic cloves, minced
- 1 tsp smoked paprika
- 1 tsp oregano
- 1/4 tsp black pepper
- Lime wedges for garnish

**Instructions:**

1. Preheat grill to medium-high heat.
2. In a bowl, mix olive oil, lime juice, minced garlic, smoked paprika, oregano, and black pepper.
3. Score the snapper on both sides and brush with the marinade.
4. Grill the snapper for 6-8 minutes per side, or until the fish is cooked through and flakes easily.
5. Serve with lime wedges.

**Nutrition Info (per serving):**

- Calories: 250
- Protein: 30g
- Carbohydrates: 2g
- Fat: 14g
- Fiber: 1g
- Sugar: 0g

**Serves:**

4

**Cooking Time:**

20 minutes

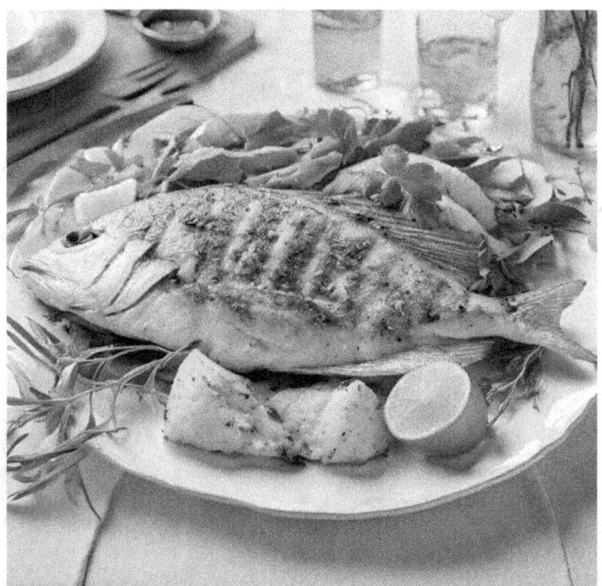

## 9. Mussels in Lemongrass Broth

**Ingredients:**

- 2 lbs mussels, cleaned and debearded
- 2 tbsp olive oil
- 2 garlic cloves, minced
- 2 stalks lemongrass, chopped
- 1 inch ginger, sliced
- 1 cup coconut milk
- 1 cup vegetable broth
- 1/4 cup lime juice
- 1/4 cup fresh cilantro, chopped

**Instructions:**

1. Heat olive oil in a large pot over medium heat.
2. Add garlic, lemongrass, and ginger, cooking for 2-3 minutes until fragrant.
3. Add coconut milk, vegetable broth, and lime juice, bringing to a simmer.
4. Add mussels, cover, and cook for 5-7 minutes, or until mussels open.
5. Discard any unopened mussels.
6. Garnish with fresh cilantro and serve immediately.

**Nutrition Info (per serving):**

- Calories: 250
- Protein: 18g
- Carbohydrates: 7g
- Fat: 16g
- Fiber: 2g
- Sugar: 3g

**Serves:**

4

**Cooking Time:**

15 minutes

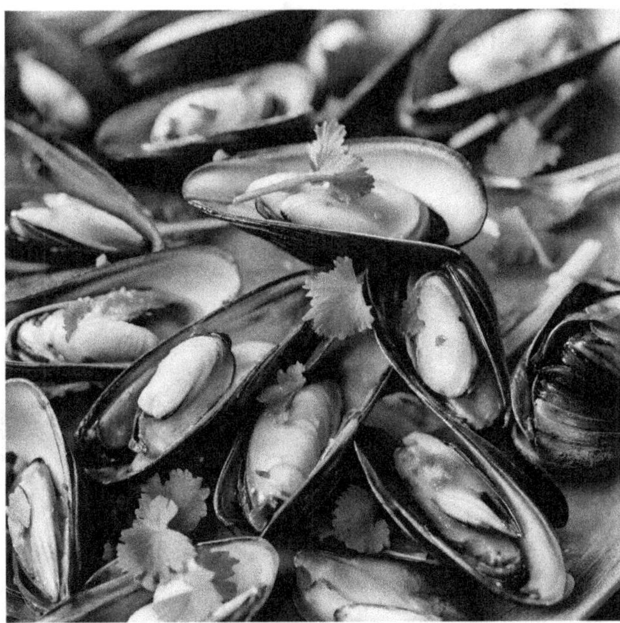

## 10. Swordfish Kebabs with Vegetables

**Ingredients:**

- 1 lb swordfish, cut into 1-inch cubes
- 1 red bell pepper, cut into 1-inch pieces
- 1 yellow bell pepper, cut into 1-inch pieces
- 1 zucchini, sliced
- 1 red onion, cut into wedges
- 2 tbsp olive oil
- 1 tbsp lemon juice
- 1 tsp oregano
- 1/4 tsp black pepper

**Instructions:**

1. Preheat grill to medium-high heat.
2. In a bowl, mix olive oil, lemon juice, oregano, and black pepper.
3. Thread swordfish cubes, bell peppers, zucchini, and red onion onto skewers.
4. Brush kebabs with the olive oil mixture.
5. Grill kebabs for 10-12 minutes, turning occasionally, until the swordfish is cooked through and vegetables are tender.
6. Serve immediately.

**Nutrition Info (per serving):**

- Calories: 250
- Protein: 25g
- Carbohydrates: 10g
- Fat: 12g
- Fiber: 3g
- Sugar: 5g

**Serves:**

4

**Cooking Time:**

20 minutes

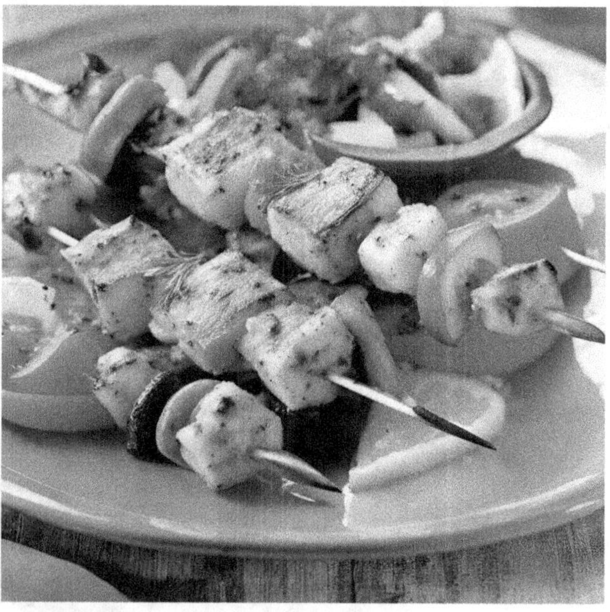

**11. Flounder with Parsley and Garlic Butter**
**Ingredients:**

- 4 flounder fillets
- 3 tbsp olive oil
- 2 garlic cloves, minced
- 1/4 cup fresh parsley, chopped
- 1 lemon, juiced
- Lemon slices for garnish

**Instructions:**

1. Heat olive oil in a large skillet over medium heat.
2. Add minced garlic and cook for 1-2 minutes until fragrant.
3. Add flounder fillets and cook for 3-4 minutes per side, until the fish is golden brown and cooked through.
4. Remove from heat and drizzle with lemon juice.
5. Sprinkle with fresh parsley and garnish with lemon slices.
6. Serve immediately.

**Nutrition Info (per serving):**

- Calories: 210
- Protein: 23g
- Carbohydrates: 2g
- Fat: 12g
- Fiber: 1g
- Sugar: 1g

**Serves:**

4

**Cooking Time:**

15 minutes

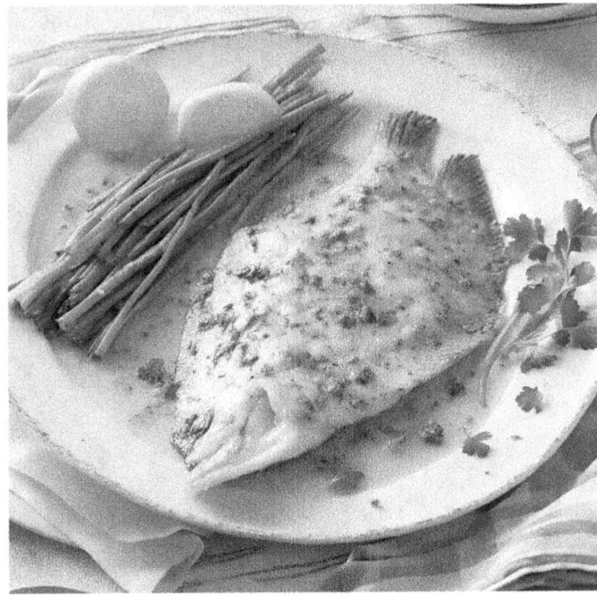

## 12. Scallop Ceviche with Avocado

**Ingredients:**

- 1 lb fresh scallops, diced
- 1/2 cup lime juice
- 1/4 cup lemon juice
- 1 avocado, diced
- 1/2 cup red onion, finely chopped
- 1/2 cup fresh cilantro, chopped
- 1 jalapeño, seeded and minced
- 1 garlic clove, minced
- 1/4 tsp black pepper

**Instructions:**

1. In a glass bowl, combine the scallops, lime juice, and lemon juice. Cover and refrigerate for 1 hour until the scallops are opaque.
2. Drain the scallops, then mix in the avocado, red onion, cilantro, jalapeño, minced garlic, and black pepper.
3. Serve immediately or chill for up to 1 hour before serving.

**Nutrition Info (per serving):**

- Calories: 180
- Protein: 18g
- Carbohydrates: 9g
- Fat: 8g
- Fiber: 4g
- Sugar: 2g

**Serves:**

4

**Cooking Time:**

1 hour 15 minutes

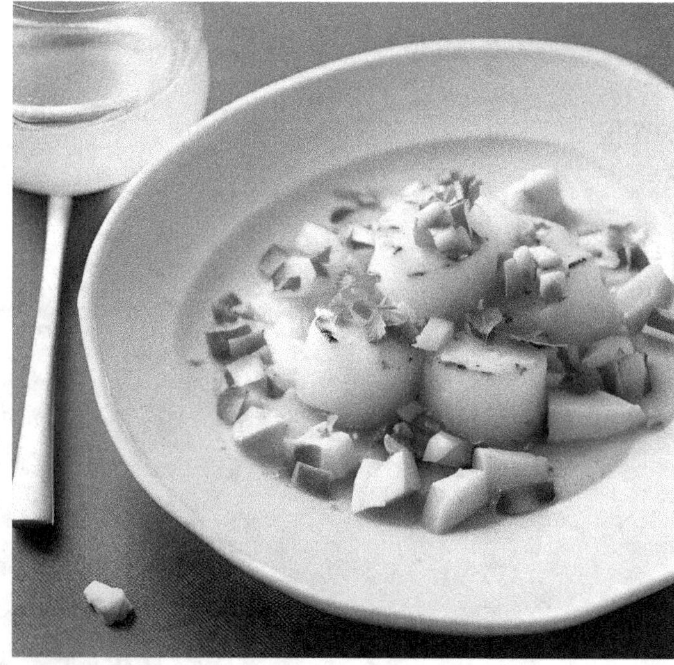

## 13. Monkfish Medallions with Herb Sauce

**Ingredients:**

- 1 lb monkfish fillets, cut into medallions
- 2 tbsp olive oil
- 1/2 cup chicken broth (low sodium)
- 1/4 cup white wine
- 1 tbsp lemon juice
- 2 garlic cloves, minced
- 1/4 cup fresh parsley, chopped
- 1/4 tsp black pepper

**Instructions:**

1. Heat olive oil in a large skillet over medium-high heat.
2. Add the monkfish medallions and cook for 3-4 minutes per side until golden brown and cooked through. Remove from skillet and set aside.
3. In the same skillet, add garlic and cook for 1 minute until fragrant.
4. Add chicken broth, white wine, and lemon juice, stirring to combine.
5. Simmer for 2-3 minutes until slightly reduced.
6. Return monkfish to the skillet, spooning the sauce over the medallions.
7. Garnish with fresh parsley and black pepper, then serve immediately.

**Nutrition Info (per serving):**

- Calories: 220
- Protein: 24g
- Carbohydrates: 2g
- Fat: 10g
- Fiber: 1g
- Sugar: 0g

**Serves:**

4

**Cooking Time:**

20 minutes

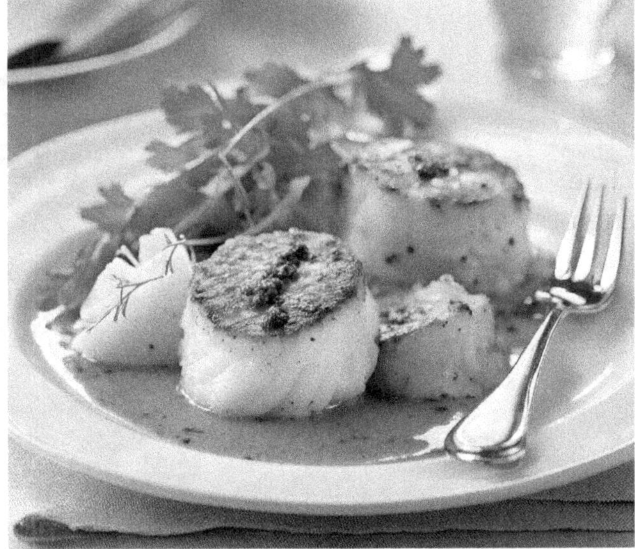

**14. Shrimp Gazpacho**
**Ingredients:**

- 1 lb shrimp, peeled and deveined
- 4 tomatoes, chopped
- 1 cucumber, peeled and diced
- 1 red bell pepper, diced
- 1 small red onion, finely chopped
- 2 garlic cloves, minced
- 1/4 cup red wine vinegar
- 1/4 cup olive oil
- 1 cup tomato juice
- 1 tbsp fresh basil, chopped

**Instructions:**

1. Bring a pot of water to a boil and cook the shrimp until pink, about 2-3 minutes. Drain and set aside to cool.
2. In a large bowl, combine the tomatoes, cucumber, red bell pepper, red onion, and garlic.
3. Add the red wine vinegar, olive oil, tomato juice, and basil, stirring to combine.
4. Stir in the cooled shrimp.
5. Chill the gazpacho in the refrigerator for at least 1 hour before serving.

**Nutrition Info (per serving):**

- Calories: 200
- Protein: 18g
- Carbohydrates: 12g
- Fat: 10g
- Fiber: 3g
- Sugar: 7g

**Serves:**

4

**Cooking Time:**

1 hour 20 minutes

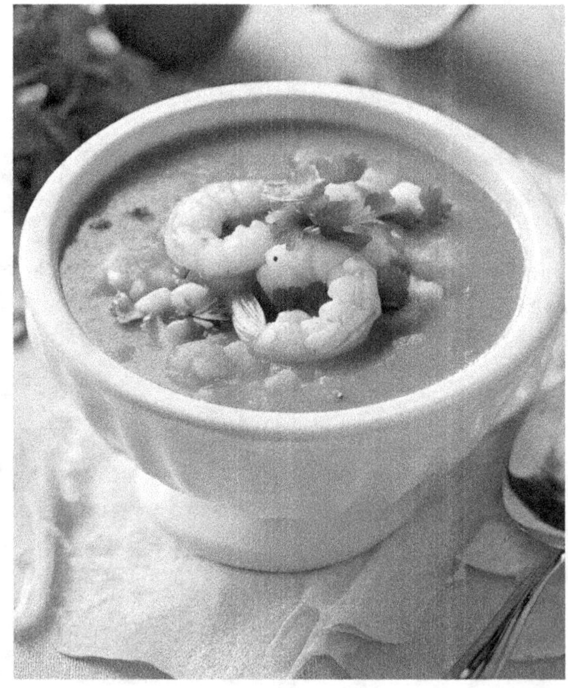

## 15. Catfish in Tomato Basil Sauce

**Ingredients:**

- 4 catfish fillets
- 2 tbsp olive oil
- 1 onion, chopped
- 3 garlic cloves, minced
- 4 tomatoes, chopped
- 1/4 cup tomato paste
- 1/2 cup vegetable broth
- 1/4 cup fresh basil, chopped
- 1/4 tsp black pepper

**Instructions:**

1. Heat olive oil in a large skillet over medium heat.
2. Add onion and garlic, cooking until softened, about 5 minutes.
3. Add tomatoes, tomato paste, and vegetable broth, stirring to combine.
4. Simmer for 10 minutes until the sauce thickens.
5. Add catfish fillets to the skillet, spooning the sauce over the fish.
6. Cover and cook for 10-12 minutes, or until the fish is cooked through.
7. Garnish with fresh basil and black pepper, then serve.

**Nutrition Info (per serving):**

- Calories: 300
- Protein: 28g
- Carbohydrates: 10g
- Fat: 15g
- Fiber: 3g
- Sugar: 6g

**Serves:**

4

**Cooking Time:**

30 minutes

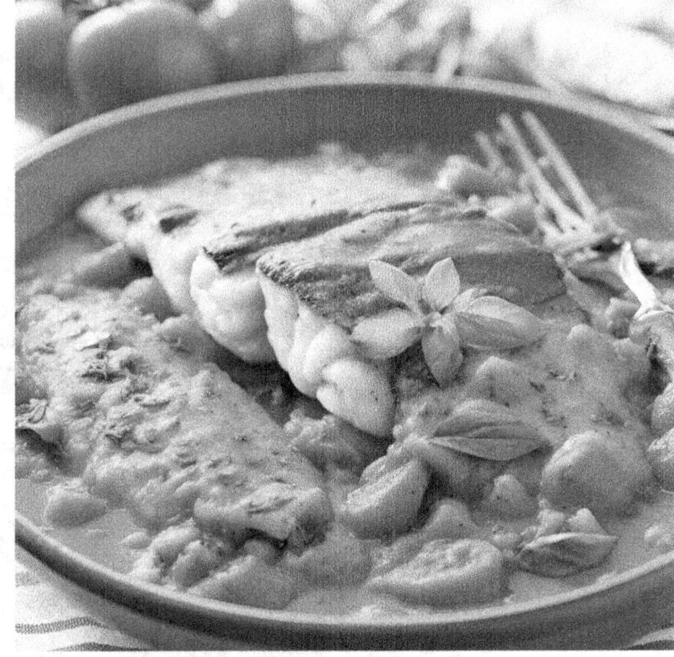

**16. Anchovies Marinated in Vinegar**

**Ingredients:**

- 1 lb fresh anchovies, cleaned and filleted
- 1 cup white wine vinegar
- 1/2 cup water
- 2 garlic cloves, thinly sliced
- 1/4 cup fresh parsley, chopped
- 1/4 tsp red pepper flakes (optional)
- 1/4 cup olive oil

**Instructions:**

1. In a bowl, combine white wine vinegar and water.
2. Add the anchovy fillets and let marinate in the refrigerator for 1-2 hours until the fillets turn white.
3. Drain the anchovies and arrange them on a serving plate.
4. Sprinkle with garlic slices, fresh parsley, and red pepper flakes (if using).
5. Drizzle with olive oil and serve.

**Nutrition Info (per serving):**

- Calories: 180
- Protein: 15g
- Carbohydrates: 1g
- Fat: 13g
- Fiber: 1g
- Sugar: 0g

**Serves:**

4

**Cooking Time:**

2 hours 10 minutes

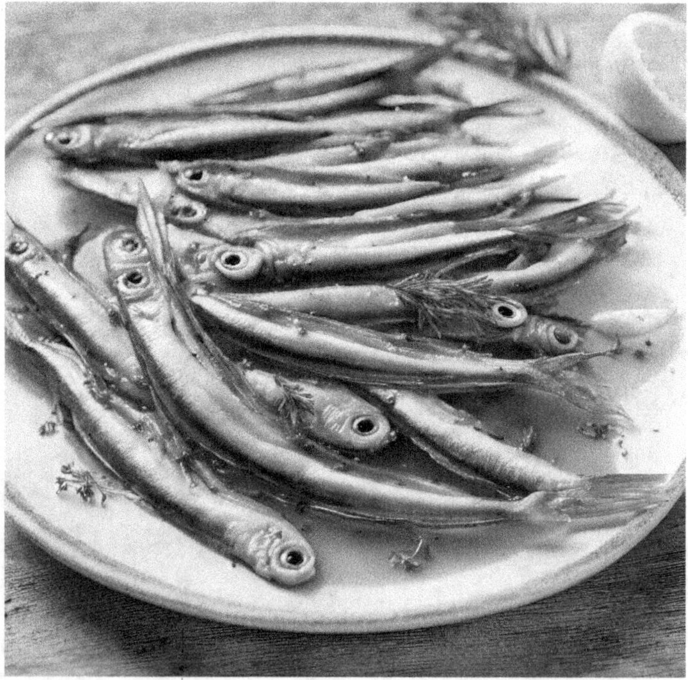

## 17. Pan-Seared Branzino with Capers

**Ingredients:**

- 4 branzino fillets
- 3 tbsp olive oil
- 1/4 cup capers, rinsed
- 2 garlic cloves, minced
- 1 lemon, juiced
- 1/4 cup fresh parsley, chopped

**Instructions:**

1. Heat 2 tbsp olive oil in a large skillet over medium-high heat.
2. Add the branzino fillets, skin-side down, and cook for 3-4 minutes until the skin is crispy.
3. Flip the fillets and cook for another 2-3 minutes until the fish is cooked through.
4. Remove the fish from the skillet and set aside.
5. Add the remaining olive oil, capers, and minced garlic to the skillet. Cook for 1-2 minutes until fragrant.
6. Stir in the lemon juice and fresh parsley.
7. Pour the sauce over the branzino fillets and serve immediately.

**Nutrition Info (per serving):**

- Calories: 250
- Protein: 26g
- Carbohydrates: 3g
- Fat: 15g
- Fiber: 1g
- Sugar: 0g

**Serves:**

4

**Cooking Time:**

15 minutes

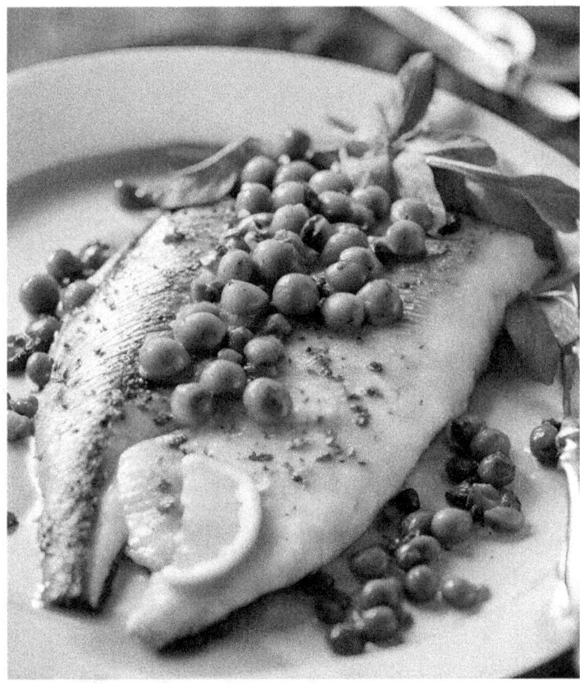

**18. Octopus Carpaccio with Olive Oil and Lemon**

**Ingredients:**

- 1 lb cooked octopus, thinly sliced
- 1/4 cup extra-virgin olive oil
- 2 tbsp lemon juice
- 1 garlic clove, minced
- 1/4 tsp red pepper flakes (optional)
- 2 tbsp fresh parsley, chopped

**Instructions:**

1. Arrange the thinly sliced octopus on a serving platter.
2. In a small bowl, mix the olive oil, lemon juice, minced garlic, and red pepper flakes (if using).
3. Drizzle the olive oil mixture over the octopus slices.
4. Sprinkle with fresh parsley.
5. Serve immediately or chill for 30 minutes before serving.

**Nutrition Info (per serving):**

- Calories: 200
- Protein: 20g
- Carbohydrates: 2g
- Fat: 13g
- Fiber: 1g
- Sugar: 0g

**Serves:**

4

**Cooking Time:**

10 minutes (plus optional chilling time)

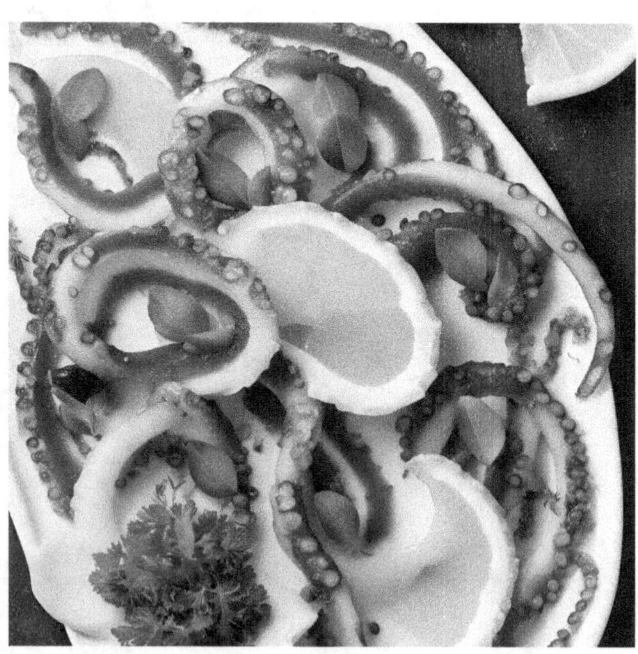

## 19. Haddock Baked with Mustard and Herbs

**Ingredients:**

- 4 haddock fillets
- 2 tbsp Dijon mustard
- 2 tbsp olive oil
- 1 tbsp lemon juice
- 1 tbsp fresh dill, chopped
- 1 tbsp fresh thyme, chopped
- 1/4 tsp black pepper

**Instructions:**

1. Preheat oven to 400°F (200°C).
2. In a small bowl, mix the Dijon mustard, olive oil, lemon juice, fresh dill, fresh thyme, and black pepper.
3. Place the haddock fillets on a baking sheet lined with parchment paper.
4. Brush the mustard mixture over the haddock fillets.
5. Bake for 12-15 minutes, or until the fish is cooked through and flakes easily with a fork.
6. Serve immediately.

**Nutrition Info (per serving):**

- Calories: 220
- Protein: 25g
- Carbohydrates: 2g
- Fat: 12g
- Fiber: 1g
- Sugar: 0g

**Serves:**

4

**Cooking Time:**

20 minutes

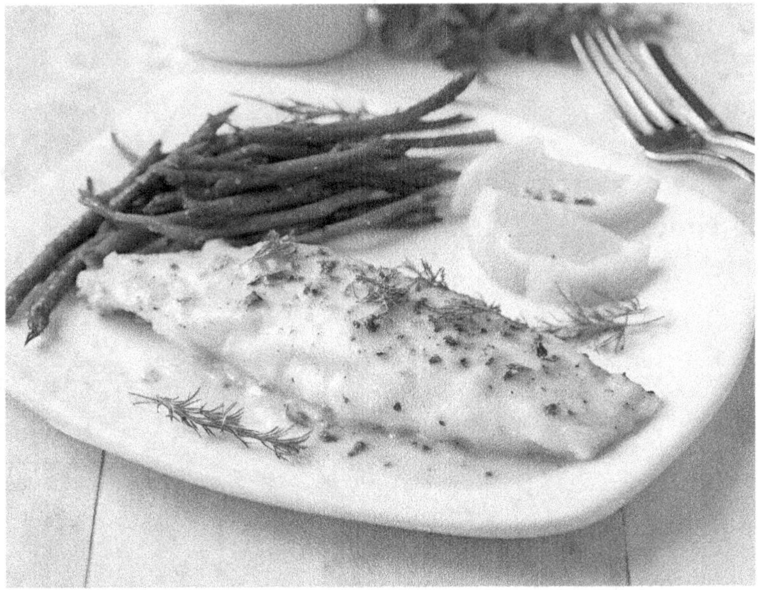

## 20. Salmon Poke Bowl with Mango and Avocado

**Ingredients:**

- 1 lb sushi-grade salmon, diced
- 1/4 cup low-sodium soy sauce
- 1 tbsp sesame oil
- 1 tbsp rice vinegar
- 1 tbsp sesame seeds
- 1 mango, diced
- 1 avocado, diced
- 1 cucumber, thinly sliced
- 1 cup cooked brown rice
- 2 tbsp fresh chives, chopped

**Instructions:**

1. In a bowl, mix the soy sauce, sesame oil, rice vinegar, and sesame seeds.
2. Add the diced salmon to the bowl and gently toss to coat. Let marinate for 10 minutes.
3. Divide the cooked brown rice between four bowls.
4. Top each bowl with the marinated salmon, diced mango, diced avocado, and cucumber slices.
5. Sprinkle with fresh chives.
6. Serve immediately.

**Nutrition Info (per serving):**

- Calories: 450
- Protein: 30g
- Carbohydrates: 35g
- Fat: 20g
- Fiber: 7g
- Sugar: 10g

**Serves:**

4

**Cooking Time:**

20 minutes

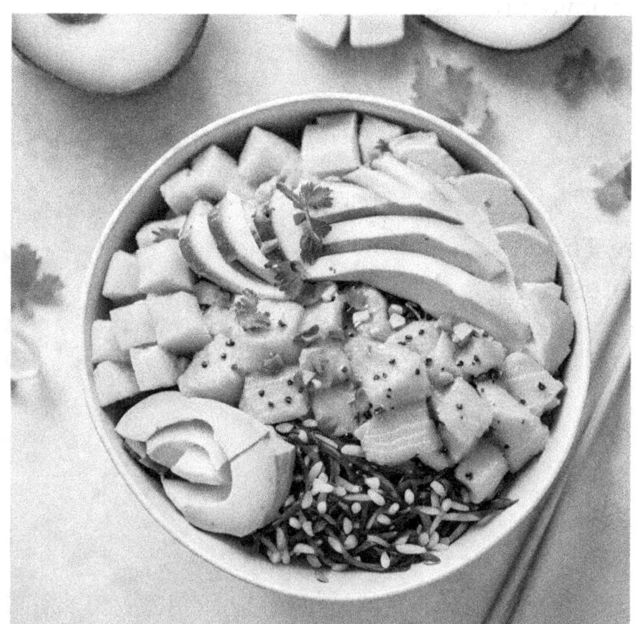

## 21. Prawn Stir-Fry with Broccoli and Bell Peppers

**Ingredients:**

- 1 lb prawns, peeled and deveined
- 2 tbsp olive oil
- 2 garlic cloves, minced
- 1 inch ginger, grated
- 2 cups broccoli florets
- 1 red bell pepper, sliced
- 1 yellow bell pepper, sliced
- 1 tbsp soy sauce (low sodium)
- 1 tbsp sesame oil
- 1 tsp sesame seeds
- 1 tbsp fresh cilantro, chopped

**Instructions:**

1. Heat olive oil in a large skillet or wok over medium-high heat.
2. Add the garlic and ginger, cooking for 1-2 minutes until fragrant.
3. Add the prawns and cook until they turn pink, about 3-4 minutes. Remove and set aside.
4. In the same skillet, add broccoli and bell peppers, stir-frying for 5-7 minutes until tender-crisp.
5. Return the prawns to the skillet, add soy sauce and sesame oil, and stir to combine.
6. Cook for an additional 2 minutes until heated through.
7. Sprinkle with sesame seeds and fresh cilantro before serving.

**Nutrition Info (per serving):**

- Calories: 250
- Protein: 25g
- Carbohydrates: 12g
- Fat: 12g
- Fiber: 4g
- Sugar: 5g

**Serves:**

4

**Cooking Time:**

20 minutes

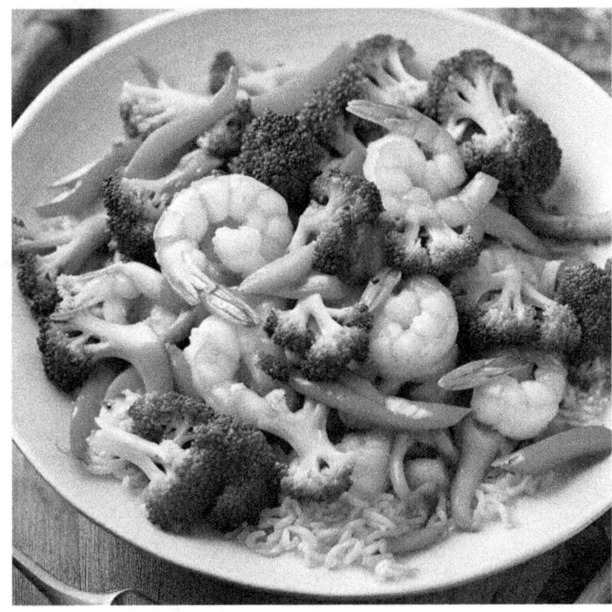

## 22. Smoked Salmon and Cucumber Rolls

**Ingredients:**

- 8 oz smoked salmon, thinly sliced
- 1 large cucumber, thinly sliced lengthwise
- 1/4 cup cream cheese (dairy-free if preferred)
- 1 tbsp fresh dill, chopped
- 1 lemon, cut into wedges

**Instructions:**

1. Spread a thin layer of cream cheese on each cucumber slice.
2. Place a slice of smoked salmon on top of the cream cheese.
3. Sprinkle with fresh dill.
4. Roll up the cucumber slices and secure with a toothpick if needed.
5. Serve with lemon wedges.

**Nutrition Info (per serving):**

- Calories: 120
- Protein: 8g
- Carbohydrates: 4g
- Fat: 8g
- Fiber: 1g
- Sugar: 2g

**Serves:**

4

**Cooking Time:**

10 minutes

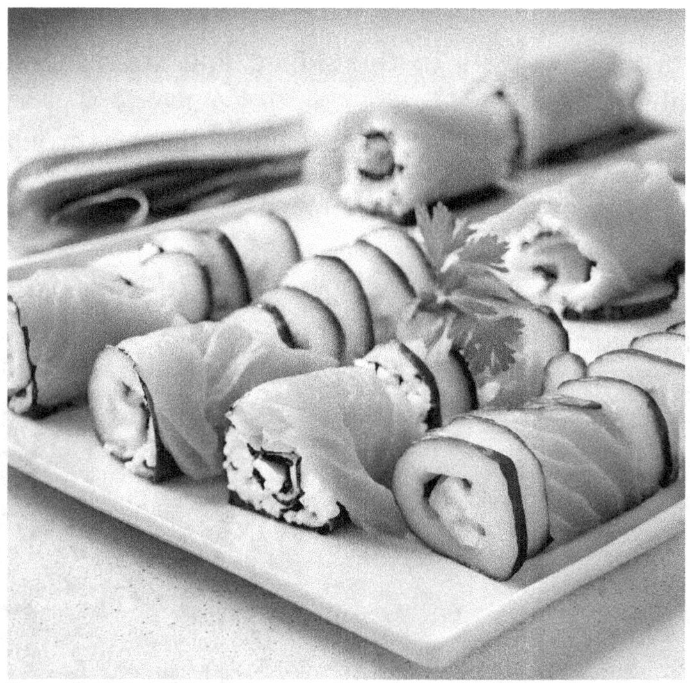

## 23. Sardines Grilled with Lemon Pepper

**Ingredients:**

- 8 fresh sardines, cleaned and gutted
- 3 tbsp olive oil
- 2 lemons, juiced and zested
- 1 tsp black pepper
- 1 tbsp fresh parsley, chopped

**Instructions:**

1. Preheat grill to medium-high heat.
2. In a bowl, mix olive oil, lemon juice, lemon zest, and black pepper.
3. Brush the sardines with the lemon pepper mixture.
4. Grill the sardines for 3-4 minutes per side, until cooked through and slightly charred.
5. Garnish with fresh parsley and serve immediately.

**Nutrition Info (per serving):**

- Calories: 200
- Protein: 20g
- Carbohydrates: 1g
- Fat: 13g
- Fiber: 1g
- Sugar: 0g

**Serves:**

4

**Cooking Time:**

15 minutes

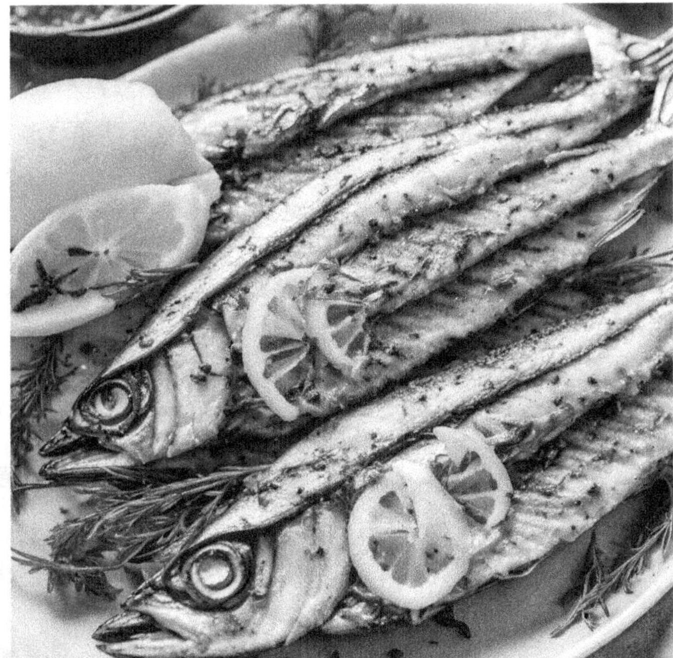

## 24. Lobster Tail Steamed with Ginger

**Ingredients:**

- 4 lobster tails
- 2 inches ginger, thinly sliced
- 2 tbsp soy sauce (low sodium)
- 1 tbsp sesame oil
- 1 tbsp fresh chives, chopped

**Instructions:**

1. Prepare a steamer or use a pot with a steamer insert.
2. Place the ginger slices in the steamer.
3. Arrange the lobster tails on top of the ginger.
4. Steam for 8-10 minutes, or until the lobster meat is opaque and cooked through.
5. In a small bowl, mix soy sauce and sesame oil.
6. Drizzle the sauce over the lobster tails.
7. Garnish with fresh chives and serve immediately.

**Nutrition Info (per serving):**

- Calories: 210
- Protein: 28g
- Carbohydrates: 2g
- Fat: 10g
- Fiber: 1g
- Sugar: 0g

**Serves:**

4

**Cooking Time:**

15 minutes

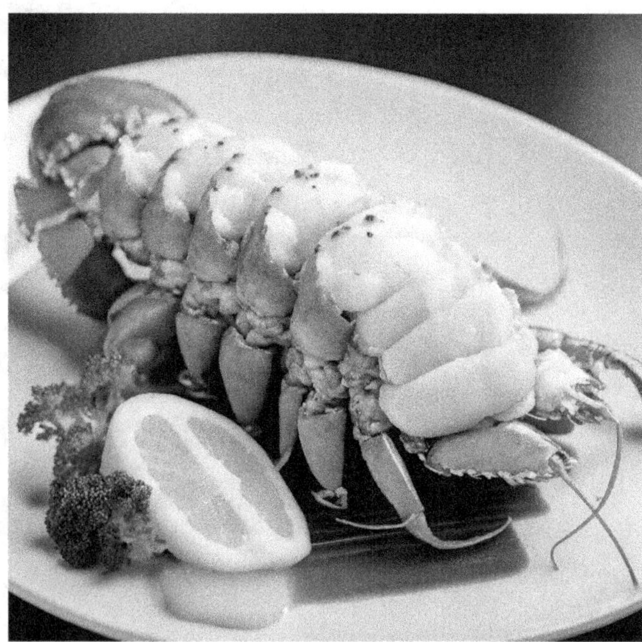

## 25. Grilled Trout with Herbs

**Ingredients:**

- 4 trout fillets
- 3 tbsp olive oil
- 1 lemon, juiced and zested
- 2 garlic cloves, minced
- 1 tbsp fresh thyme, chopped
- 1 tbsp fresh rosemary, chopped

**Instructions:**

1. Preheat grill to medium-high heat.
2. In a small bowl, mix olive oil, lemon juice, lemon zest, minced garlic, thyme, and rosemary.
3. Brush the trout fillets with the herb mixture.
4. Grill the trout fillets for 4-5 minutes per side, until the fish is cooked through and flakes easily.
5. Serve immediately.

**Nutrition Info (per serving):**

- Calories: 250
- Protein: 28g
- Carbohydrates: 2g
- Fat: 14g
- Fiber: 1g
- Sugar: 0g

**Serves:**

4

**Cooking Time:**

15 minutes

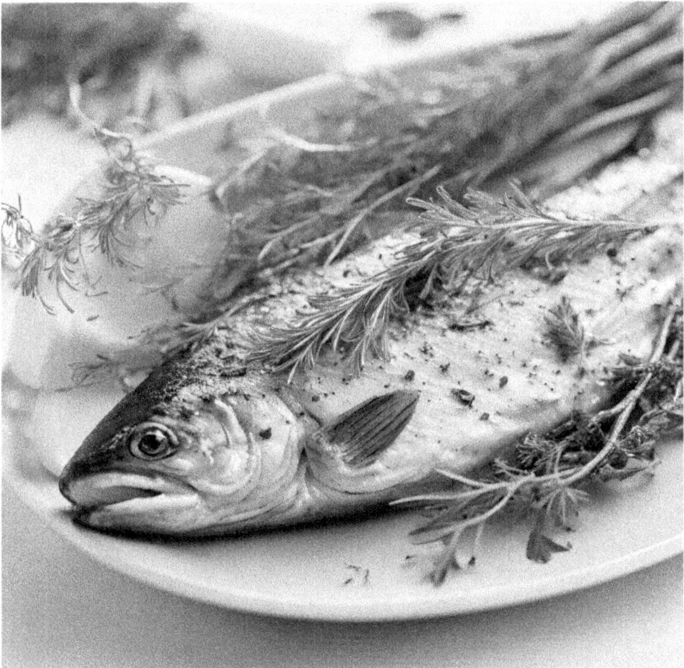

**26. Oyster Shooters with Tomato Juice**
**Ingredients:**

- 12 fresh oysters, shucked
- 1 cup tomato juice
- 2 tbsp lemon juice
- 1 tsp Worcestershire sauce
- 1/4 tsp hot sauce (optional)
- 1 tbsp fresh parsley, chopped

**Instructions:**

1. In a small bowl, mix tomato juice, lemon juice, Worcestershire sauce, and hot sauce (if using).
2. Place one oyster in each shot glass.
3. Pour the tomato juice mixture over the oysters.
4. Garnish with fresh parsley.
5. Serve immediately.

**Nutrition Info (per serving, 3 shooters):**

- Calories: 50
- Protein: 6g
- Carbohydrates: 3g
- Fat: 1g
- Fiber: 0g
- Sugar: 1g

**Serves:**
4
**Cooking Time:**
10 minutes

## 27. Mackerel Fillet with Tomato Salsa

**Ingredients:**

- 4 mackerel fillets
- 3 tbsp olive oil
- 1 lemon, juiced
- 2 cups cherry tomatoes, quartered
- 1 small red onion, finely chopped
- 1 garlic clove, minced
- 1/4 cup fresh cilantro, chopped
- 1 jalapeño, seeded and minced (optional)

**Instructions:**

1. Preheat grill to medium-high heat.
2. Brush mackerel fillets with 2 tbsp olive oil and lemon juice.
3. Grill the fillets for 3-4 minutes per side, until cooked through and flaky.
4. In a bowl, mix cherry tomatoes, red onion, garlic, cilantro, jalapeño (if using), and the remaining 1 tbsp olive oil.
5. Spoon the tomato salsa over the grilled mackerel fillets.
6. Serve immediately.

**Nutrition Info (per serving):**

- Calories: 300
- Protein: 26g
- Carbohydrates: 6g
- Fat: 20g
- Fiber: 2g
- Sugar: 4g

**Serves:**

4

**Cooking Time:**

20 minutes

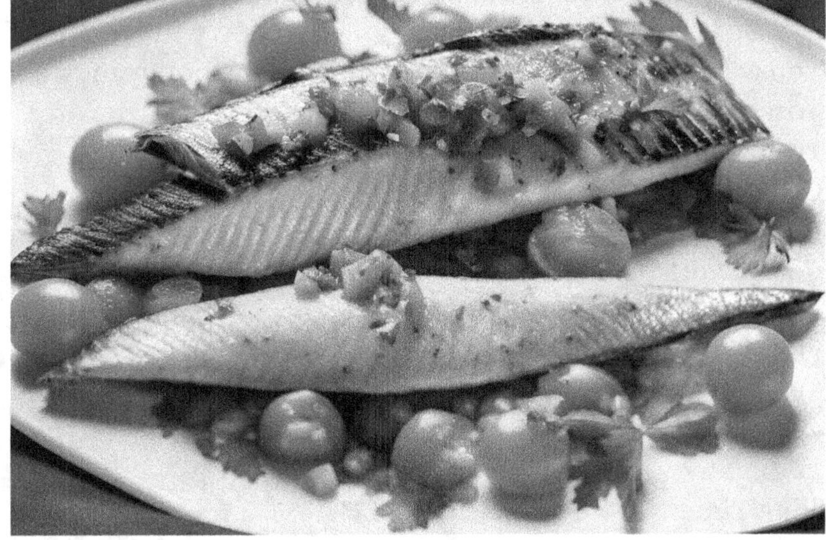

# Poultry Recipes

## 1. Honey Mustard Chicken Salad

**Ingredients:**

- 2 boneless, skinless chicken breasts
- 2 tbsp olive oil
- 2 tbsp honey
- 2 tbsp Dijon mustard
- 1 tbsp apple cider vinegar
- 4 cups mixed greens (e.g., spinach, arugula, lettuce)
- 1/2 cup cherry tomatoes, halved
- 1/4 cup red onion, thinly sliced
- 1/4 cup chopped walnuts

**Instructions:**

1. Preheat oven to 375°F (190°C).
2. Brush the chicken breasts with 1 tbsp olive oil and place them on a baking sheet.
3. Bake for 20-25 minutes, or until the chicken is cooked through and no longer pink in the center.
4. While the chicken is baking, whisk together honey, Dijon mustard, remaining olive oil, and apple cider vinegar in a small bowl to make the dressing.
5. Once the chicken is cooked, let it cool slightly, then slice it thinly.
6. In a large bowl, combine mixed greens, cherry tomatoes, red onion, and walnuts.
7. Top with sliced chicken and drizzle with the honey mustard dressing.
8. Toss gently to combine and serve immediately.

**Nutrition Info (per serving):**

- Calories: 320
- Protein: 25g
- Carbohydrates: 14g
- Fat: 18g
- Fiber: 3g
- Sugar: 10g

**Serves:**

4

**Cooking Time:**

30 minutes

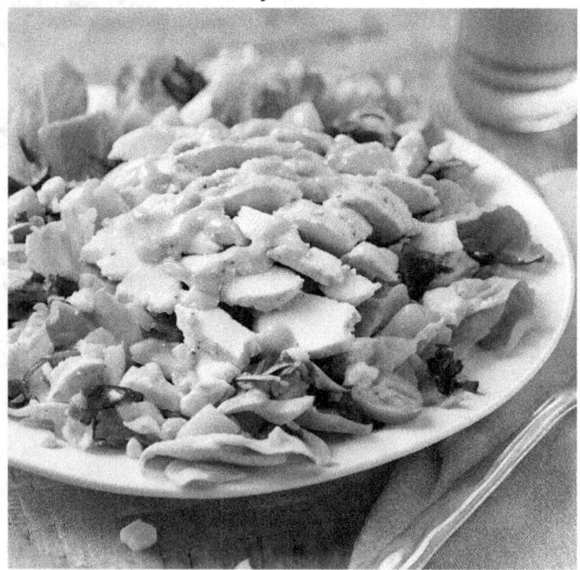

## 2. Turkey Stuffed Mushrooms

**Ingredients:**

- 12 large mushroom caps
- 1/2 lb ground turkey
- 1/4 cup almond flour
- 2 tbsp olive oil
- 1 garlic clove, minced
- 1/4 cup chopped spinach
- 1/4 tsp black pepper
- 1 tbsp fresh parsley, chopped

**Instructions:**

1. Preheat oven to 375°F (190°C).
2. Remove the stems from the mushroom caps and set aside.
3. In a skillet, heat 1 tbsp olive oil over medium heat. Add minced garlic and cook for 1-2 minutes until fragrant.
4. Add the ground turkey and cook until browned, about 5-7 minutes.
5. Stir in the almond flour, chopped spinach, and black pepper, cooking for another 2 minutes until well combined.
6. Fill each mushroom cap with the turkey mixture and place them on a baking sheet.
7. Drizzle with the remaining olive oil.
8. Bake for 15-20 minutes, or until the mushrooms are tender and the filling is golden brown.
9. Garnish with fresh parsley and serve warm.

**Nutrition Info (per serving, 3 mushrooms):**

- Calories: 150
- Protein: 10g
- Carbohydrates: 6g
- Fat: 10g
- Fiber: 2g
- Sugar: 2g

**Serves:**

4

**Cooking Time:**

25 minutes

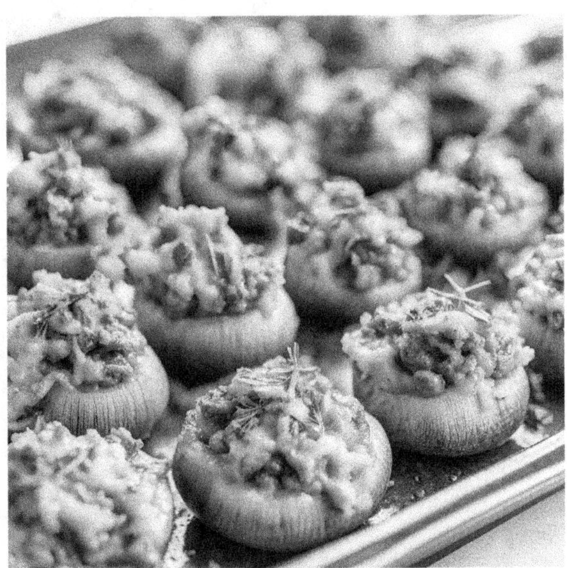

## 3. Baked Chicken with Artichokes and Capers

**Ingredients:**

- 4 boneless, skinless chicken breasts
- 1 can (14 oz) artichoke hearts, drained and quartered
- 2 tbsp capers, rinsed
- 3 tbsp olive oil
- 1 lemon, juiced and zested
- 1 garlic clove, minced
- 1/4 cup chicken broth (low sodium)
- 1 tbsp fresh parsley, chopped

**Instructions:**

1. Preheat oven to 375°F (190°C).
2. In a large baking dish, arrange the chicken breasts.
3. In a small bowl, mix olive oil, lemon juice, lemon zest, minced garlic, and chicken broth.
4. Pour the mixture over the chicken breasts.
5. Scatter the artichoke hearts and capers around the chicken.
6. Bake for 25-30 minutes, or until the chicken is cooked through and no longer pink in the center.
7. Garnish with fresh parsley before serving.

**Nutrition Info (per serving):**

- Calories: 280
- Protein: 30g
- Carbohydrates: 7g
- Fat: 14g
- Fiber: 3g
- Sugar: 2g

**Serves:**

4

**Cooking Time:**

35 minutes

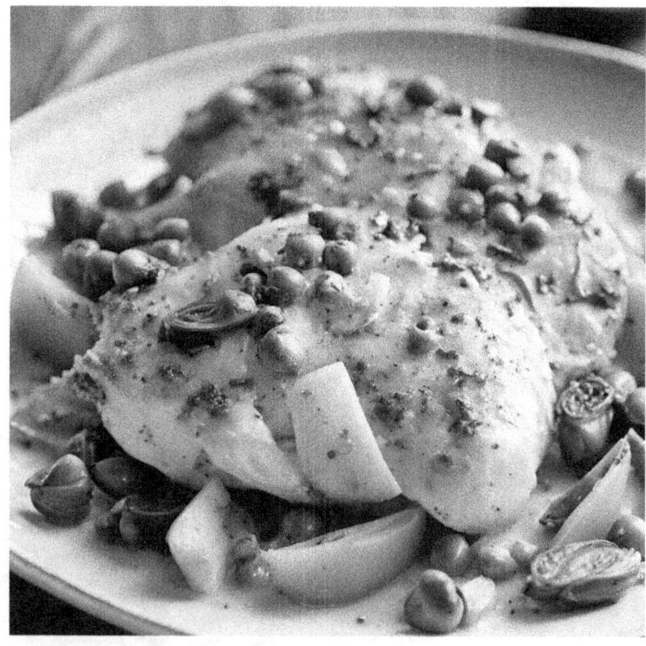

## 4. Lemon Tarragon Turkey Cutlets

**Ingredients:**

- 4 turkey cutlets
- 3 tbsp olive oil
- 1 lemon, juiced and zested
- 2 garlic cloves, minced
- 1 tbsp fresh tarragon, chopped
- 1/4 cup chicken broth (low sodium)
- 1/4 tsp black pepper

**Instructions:**

1. Heat 2 tbsp olive oil in a large skillet over medium-high heat.
2. Add the turkey cutlets and cook for 3-4 minutes per side, until golden brown and cooked through. Remove from the skillet and set aside.
3. In the same skillet, add the remaining olive oil, lemon juice, lemon zest, minced garlic, tarragon, and chicken broth.
4. Bring to a simmer and cook for 2-3 minutes until slightly reduced.
5. Return the turkey cutlets to the skillet, spooning the sauce over them.
6. Cook for an additional 2 minutes until heated through.
7. Serve immediately.

**Nutrition Info (per serving):**

- Calories: 220
- Protein: 26g
- Carbohydrates: 2g
- Fat: 12g
- Fiber: 1g
- Sugar: 0g

**Serves:**

4

**Cooking Time:**

20 minutes

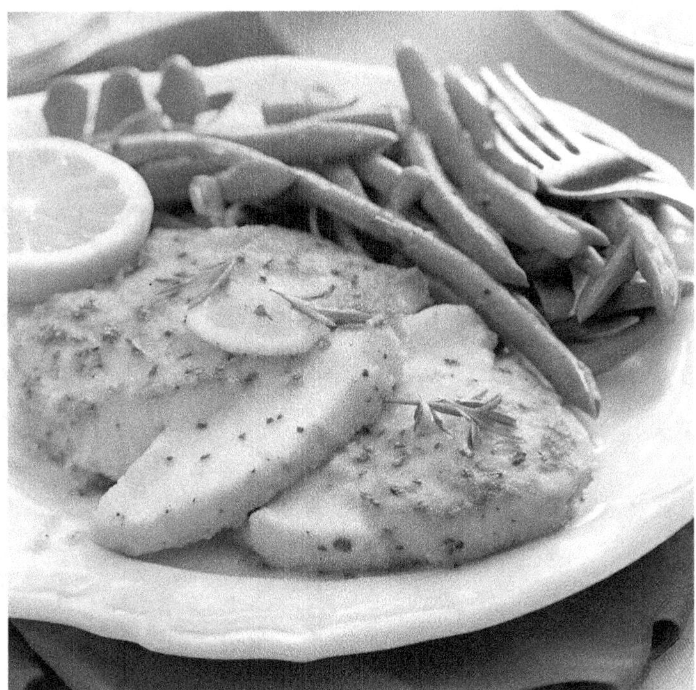

## 5. Smoked Paprika Chicken Thighs

**Ingredients:**

- 8 chicken thighs, bone-in and skin-on
- 2 tbsp olive oil
- 1 tbsp smoked paprika
- 1 tsp garlic powder
- 1 tsp onion powder
- 1 tsp dried oregano
- 1/4 tsp black pepper

**Instructions:**

1. Preheat oven to 400°F (200°C).
2. In a small bowl, mix olive oil, smoked paprika, garlic powder, onion powder, dried oregano, and black pepper.
3. Rub the spice mixture all over the chicken thighs.
4. Place the chicken thighs on a baking sheet lined with parchment paper.
5. Bake for 35-40 minutes, or until the chicken is cooked through and the skin is crispy.
6. Serve immediately.

**Nutrition Info (per serving):**

- Calories: 320
- Protein: 24g
- Carbohydrates: 2g
- Fat: 24g
- Fiber: 1g
- Sugar: 0g

**Serves:**

4

**Cooking Time:**

45 minutes

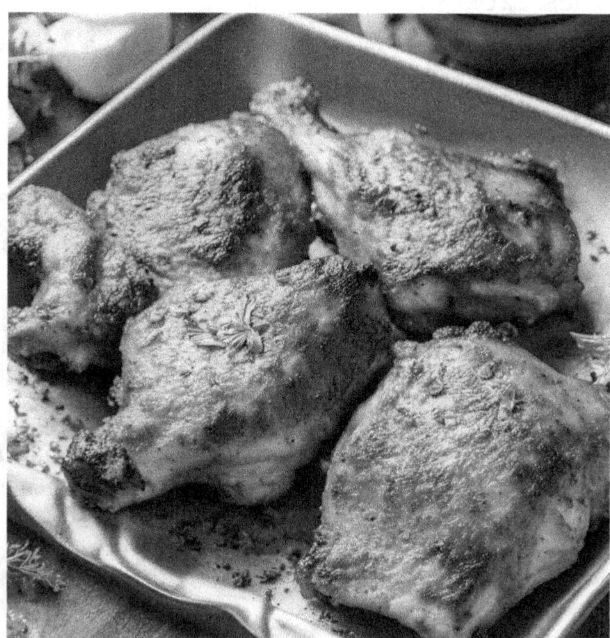

**6. Italian Herb Chicken with Roasted Vegetables**

**Ingredients:**

- 4 boneless, skinless chicken breasts
- 3 tbsp olive oil
- 1 tbsp Italian seasoning
- 1 lemon, juiced
- 1 garlic clove, minced
- 1 cup cherry tomatoes
- 1 zucchini, sliced
- 1 red bell pepper, sliced
- 1/4 tsp black pepper

**Instructions:**

1. Preheat oven to 400°F (200°C).
2. In a small bowl, mix 2 tbsp olive oil, Italian seasoning, lemon juice, minced garlic, and black pepper.
3. Rub the mixture over the chicken breasts.
4. Place the chicken breasts on a baking sheet lined with parchment paper.
5. In a large bowl, toss the cherry tomatoes, zucchini, and red bell pepper with the remaining olive oil.
6. Arrange the vegetables around the chicken on the baking sheet.
7. Bake for 25-30 minutes, or until the chicken is cooked through and the vegetables are tender.
8. Serve immediately.

**Nutrition Info (per serving):**

- Calories: 280
- Protein: 30g
- Carbohydrates: 10g
- Fat: 14g
- Fiber: 3g
- Sugar: 4g

**Serves:**

4

**Cooking Time:**

35 minutes

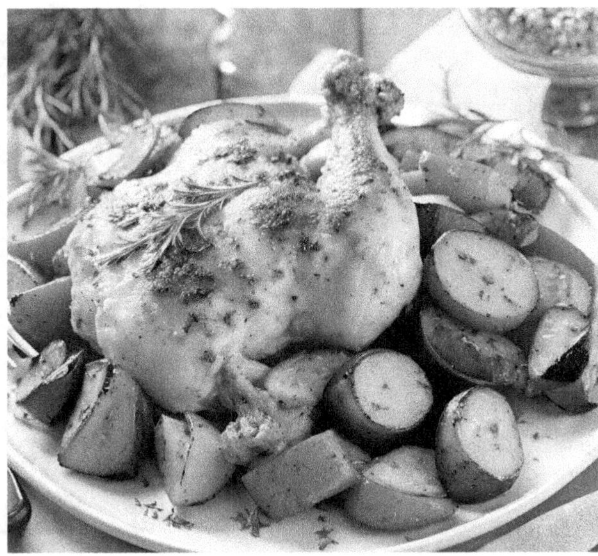

## 7. Thai Basil Chicken

**Ingredients:**

- 1 lb ground chicken
- 2 tbsp olive oil
- 1 red bell pepper, sliced
- 1 onion, sliced
- 2 garlic cloves, minced
- 1 tbsp ginger, minced
- 1/4 cup low-sodium soy sauce
- 1 tbsp fish sauce
- 1 tbsp lime juice
- 1 cup fresh basil leaves, chopped

**Instructions:**

1. Heat olive oil in a large skillet over medium-high heat.
2. Add the garlic and ginger, cooking for 1-2 minutes until fragrant.
3. Add the ground chicken and cook until browned, about 5-7 minutes.
4. Add the red bell pepper and onion, cooking for another 5 minutes until tender.
5. Stir in the soy sauce, fish sauce, and lime juice, cooking for an additional 2 minutes.
6. Remove from heat and stir in the fresh basil leaves.
7. Serve immediately over rice or quinoa.

**Nutrition Info (per serving):**

- Calories: 250
- Protein: 22g
- Carbohydrates: 10g
- Fat: 14g
- Fiber: 2g
- Sugar: 3g

**Serves:**

4

**Cooking Time:**

20 minutes

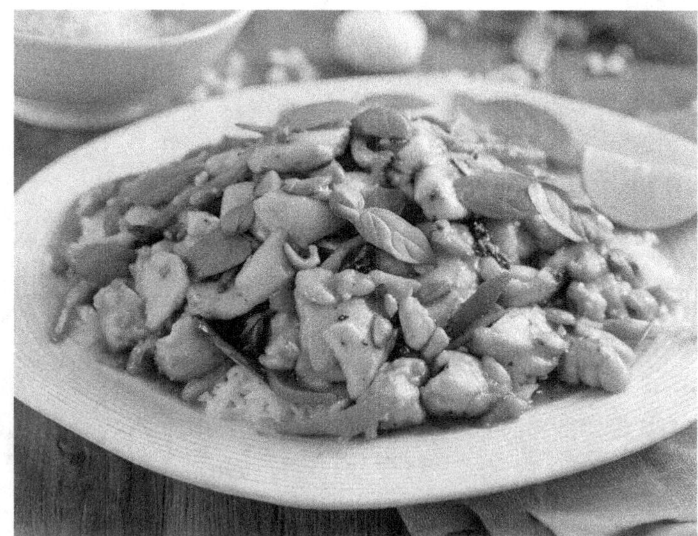

## 8. Chicken Minestrone Soup

**Ingredients:**

- 1 lb boneless, skinless chicken breasts, diced
- 2 tbsp olive oil
- 1 onion, diced
- 2 garlic cloves, minced
- 2 carrots, diced
- 2 celery stalks, diced
- 1 zucchini, diced
- 1 can (14 oz) diced tomatoes
- 4 cups chicken broth (low sodium)
- 1 cup cooked cannellini beans
- 1 tsp dried basil
- 1 tsp dried oregano
- 1/4 tsp black pepper

**Instructions:**

1. Heat olive oil in a large pot over medium heat.
2. Add the onion and garlic, cooking until softened, about 5 minutes.
3. Add the chicken and cook until browned, about 5-7 minutes.
4. Stir in the carrots, celery, and zucchini, cooking for another 5 minutes.
5. Add the diced tomatoes, chicken broth, cannellini beans, dried basil, dried oregano, and black pepper.
6. Bring to a boil, then reduce heat and simmer for 20-25 minutes until the vegetables are tender and the chicken is cooked through.
7. Serve hot.

**Nutrition Info (per serving):**

- Calories: 220
- Protein: 22g
- Carbohydrates: 20g
- Fat: 8g
- Fiber: 5g
- Sugar: 6g

**Serves:**

6

**Cooking Time:**

40 minutes

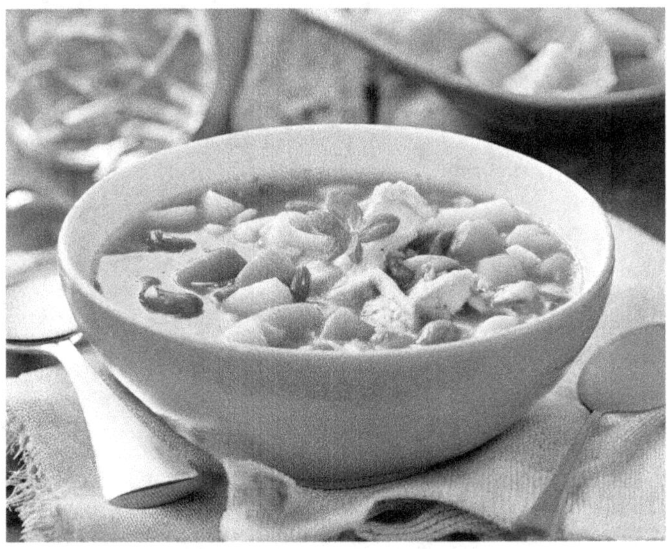

**9. Roasted Duck with Orange Sauce**

**Ingredients:**

- 1 whole duck (about 4 lbs)
- 2 tbsp olive oil
- 1/4 cup orange juice
- 1/4 cup chicken broth (low sodium)
- 2 tbsp honey
- 1 tbsp orange zest
- 2 garlic cloves, minced
- 1 tsp dried thyme

**Instructions:**

1. Preheat oven to 375°F (190°C).
2. Rub the duck with olive oil and place it in a roasting pan.
3. In a small bowl, mix orange juice, chicken broth, honey, orange zest, minced garlic, and dried thyme.
4. Pour the mixture over the duck.
5. Roast the duck for 1 hour and 30 minutes, basting every 30 minutes with the pan juices, until the duck is golden brown and the internal temperature reaches 165°F (74°C).
6. Let the duck rest for 10 minutes before carving.
7. Serve with the orange sauce from the pan.

**Nutrition Info (per serving):**

- Calories: 450
- Protein: 28g
- Carbohydrates: 10g
- Fat: 34g
- Fiber: 1g
- Sugar: 8g

**Serves:**

6

**Cooking Time:**

1 hour 40 minutes

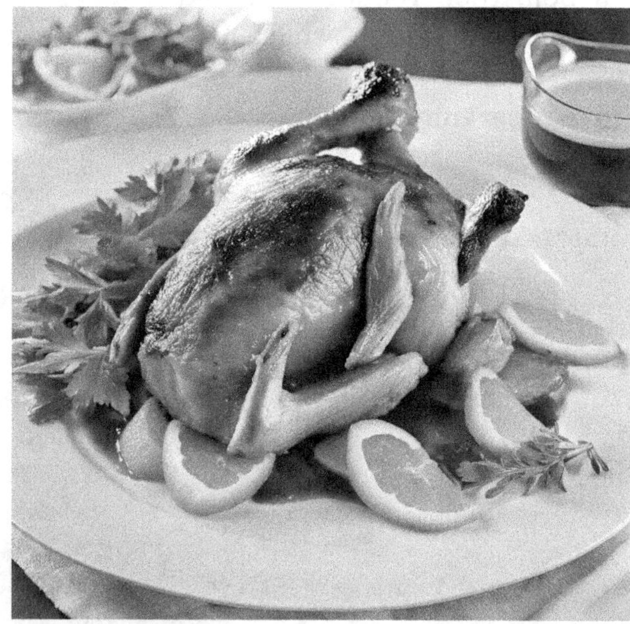

## 10. Chicken Fajitas with Bell Peppers and Onions

**Ingredients:**

- 1 lb boneless, skinless chicken breasts, sliced
- 3 tbsp olive oil
- 1 red bell pepper, sliced
- 1 green bell pepper, sliced
- 1 yellow bell pepper, sliced
- 1 onion, sliced
- 1 tsp cumin
- 1 tsp chili powder
- 1/4 tsp black pepper
- 8 small whole grain tortillas

**Instructions:**

1. Heat 2 tbsp olive oil in a large skillet over medium-high heat.
2. Add the sliced chicken, cumin, chili powder, and black pepper. Cook until the chicken is browned and cooked through, about 7-8 minutes.
3. Remove the chicken from the skillet and set aside.
4. In the same skillet, add the remaining olive oil, bell peppers, and onion. Cook until the vegetables are tender, about 5-7 minutes.
5. Return the chicken to the skillet and stir to combine with the vegetables.
6. Serve the chicken and vegetables with whole grain tortillas.

**Nutrition Info (per serving):**

- Calories: 280
- Protein: 22g
- Carbohydrates: 24g
- Fat: 10g
- Fiber: 4g
- Sugar: 4g

**Serves:**

4

**Cooking Time:**

20 minutes

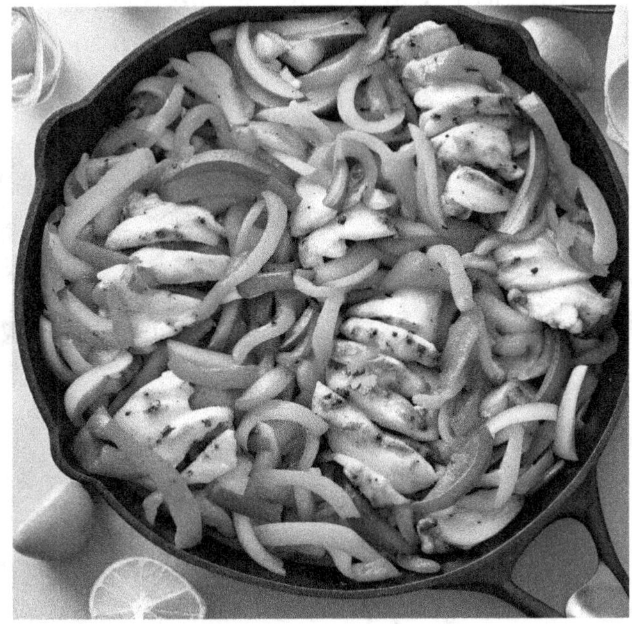

## 11. Chicken Tacos with Pineapple Salsa

**Ingredients:**

**For the chicken:**

- 1 lb boneless, skinless chicken breasts, diced
- 2 tbsp olive oil
- 1 tsp cumin
- 1 tsp paprika
- 1/4 tsp black pepper

**For the pineapple salsa:**

- 1 cup pineapple, diced
- 1/2 red onion, finely chopped
- 1 jalapeño, seeded and minced
- 1/4 cup fresh cilantro, chopped
- 1 lime, juiced

**To serve:**

- 8 small corn tortillas

**Instructions:**

1. Heat olive oil in a large skillet over medium-high heat.
2. Add the diced chicken, cumin, paprika, and black pepper. Cook until the chicken is browned and cooked through, about 7-8 minutes.
3. In a bowl, combine the diced pineapple, red onion, jalapeño, cilantro, and lime juice to make the salsa.
4. Warm the corn tortillas in a skillet or microwave.
5. Serve the chicken in the tortillas, topped with the pineapple salsa.

**Nutrition Info (per serving):**

- Calories: 250
- Protein: 20g
- Carbohydrates: 24g
- Fat: 8g
- Fiber: 3g
- Sugar: 6g

**Serves:**

4

**Cooking Time:**

20 minutes

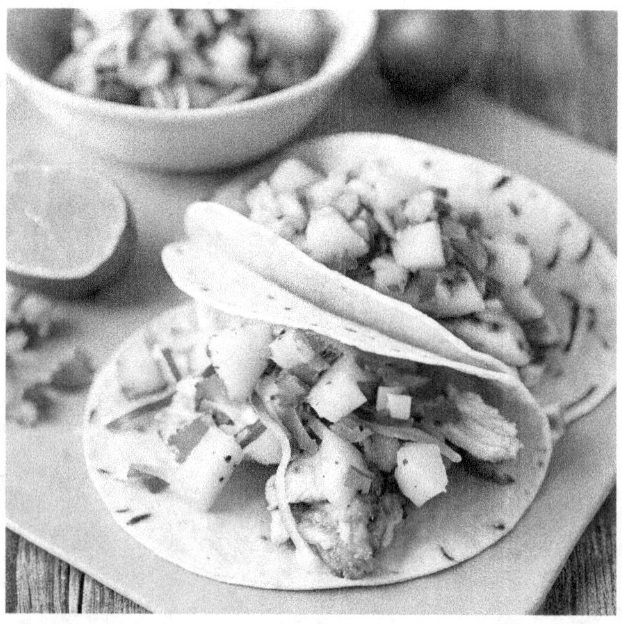

**12. Garlic and Herb Chicken Drumsticks**

**Ingredients:**

- 8 chicken drumsticks
- 3 tbsp olive oil
- 4 garlic cloves, minced
- 1 tbsp dried oregano
- 1 tbsp dried thyme
- 1 lemon, juiced and zested

**Instructions:**

1. Preheat oven to 400°F (200°C).
2. In a small bowl, mix olive oil, minced garlic, dried oregano, dried thyme, lemon juice, and lemon zest.
3. Rub the mixture all over the chicken drumsticks.
4. Place the drumsticks on a baking sheet lined with parchment paper.
5. Bake for 35-40 minutes, or until the chicken is cooked through and the skin is crispy.
6. Serve immediately.

**Nutrition Info (per serving):**

- Calories: 320
- Protein: 24g
- Carbohydrates: 2g
- Fat: 24g
- Fiber: 1g
- Sugar: 0g

**Serves:**

4

**Cooking Time:**

45 minutes

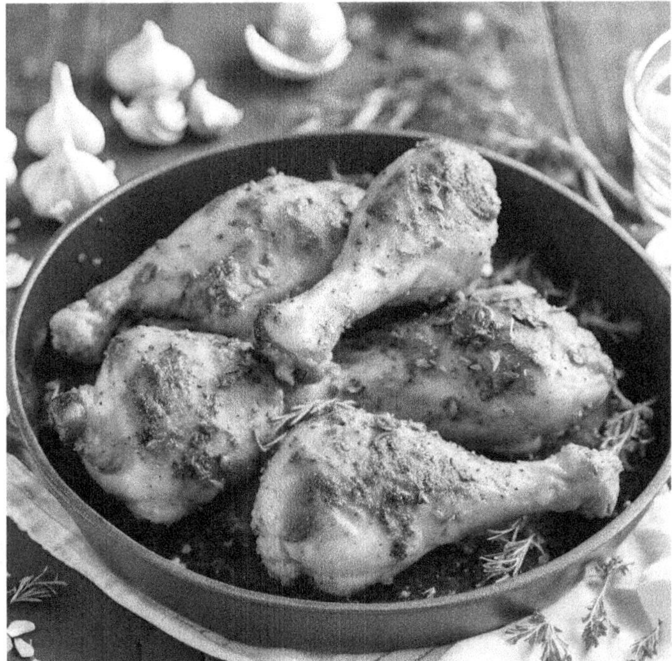

## 13. Chicken Curry with Coconut Milk

**Ingredients:**

- 1 lb boneless, skinless chicken breasts, diced
- 2 tbsp olive oil
- 1 onion, chopped
- 3 garlic cloves, minced
- 1 tbsp ginger, minced
- 2 tbsp curry powder
- 1 can (14 oz) coconut milk
- 1 cup chicken broth (low sodium)
- 1 cup diced tomatoes
- 1 cup chopped spinach
- 1/4 cup fresh cilantro, chopped

**Instructions:**

1. Heat olive oil in a large pot over medium heat.
2. Add the onion, garlic, and ginger, cooking until softened, about 5 minutes.
3. Add the diced chicken and curry powder, cooking until the chicken is browned, about 5-7 minutes.
4. Stir in the coconut milk, chicken broth, and diced tomatoes.
5. Bring to a boil, then reduce heat and simmer for 20 minutes.
6. Add the chopped spinach and cook for another 5 minutes until wilted.
7. Garnish with fresh cilantro and serve hot.

**Nutrition Info (per serving):**

- Calories: 350
- Protein: 25g
- Carbohydrates: 10g
- Fat: 24g
- Fiber: 3g
- Sugar: 4g

**Serves:**

4

**Cooking Time:**

40 minutes

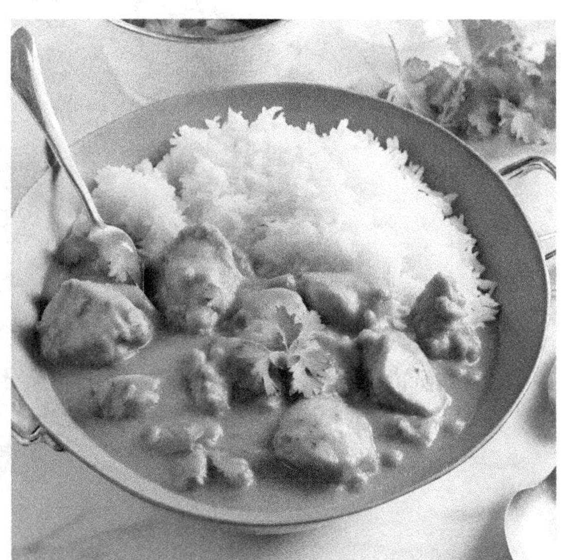

**14. Turkey Bolognese with Zucchini Noodles**

**Ingredients:**

- 1 lb ground turkey
- 2 tbsp olive oil
- 1 onion, chopped
- 3 garlic cloves, minced
- 1 carrot, diced
- 2 celery stalks, diced
- 1 can (14 oz) diced tomatoes
- 1/4 cup tomato paste
- 1 tsp dried basil
- 1 tsp dried oregano
- 1/4 tsp black pepper
- 4 large zucchinis, spiralized into noodles

**Instructions:**

1. Heat olive oil in a large skillet over medium heat.
2. Add the onion and garlic, cooking until softened, about 5 minutes.
3. Add the ground turkey, cooking until browned, about 7-8 minutes.
4. Stir in the carrot, celery, diced tomatoes, tomato paste, dried basil, dried oregano, and black pepper.
5. Simmer for 20-25 minutes until the sauce thickens.
6. In another skillet, lightly sauté the zucchini noodles for 2-3 minutes until tender.
7. Serve the turkey Bolognese over the zucchini noodles.

**Nutrition Info (per serving):**

- Calories: 280
- Protein: 26g
- Carbohydrates: 14g
- Fat: 14g
- Fiber: 4g
- Sugar: 8g

**Serves:**

4

**Cooking Time:**

40 minutes

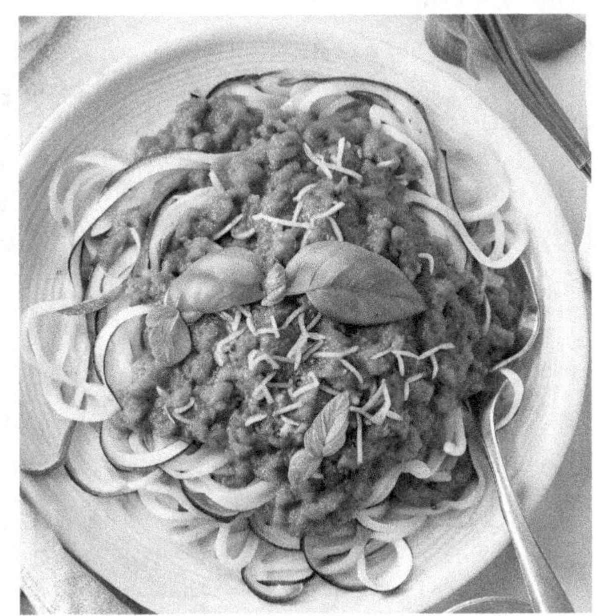

## 15. Moroccan Chicken Tagine

**Ingredients:**

- 1 lb boneless, skinless chicken thighs, diced
- 2 tbsp olive oil
- 1 onion, chopped
- 3 garlic cloves, minced
- 1 tsp ground cumin
- 1 tsp ground cinnamon
- 1 tsp ground ginger
- 1/2 tsp ground turmeric
- 1 cup chicken broth (low sodium)
- 1 can (14 oz) diced tomatoes
- 1/2 cup dried apricots, chopped
- 1/4 cup sliced almonds
- 1/4 cup fresh cilantro, chopped

**Instructions:**

1. Heat olive oil in a large pot or tagine over medium heat.
2. Add the onion and garlic, cooking until softened, about 5 minutes.
3. Add the diced chicken, ground cumin, ground cinnamon, ground ginger, and ground turmeric, cooking until the chicken is browned, about 7-8 minutes.
4. Stir in the chicken broth, diced tomatoes, and dried apricots.
5. Bring to a boil, then reduce heat and simmer for 25-30 minutes until the chicken is cooked through and the sauce thickens.
6. Garnish with sliced almonds and fresh cilantro before serving.

**Nutrition Info (per serving):**

- Calories: 320
- Protein: 24g
- Carbohydrates: 20g
- Fat: 16g
- Fiber: 5g
- Sugar: 10g

**Serves:**

4

**Cooking Time:**

40 minutes

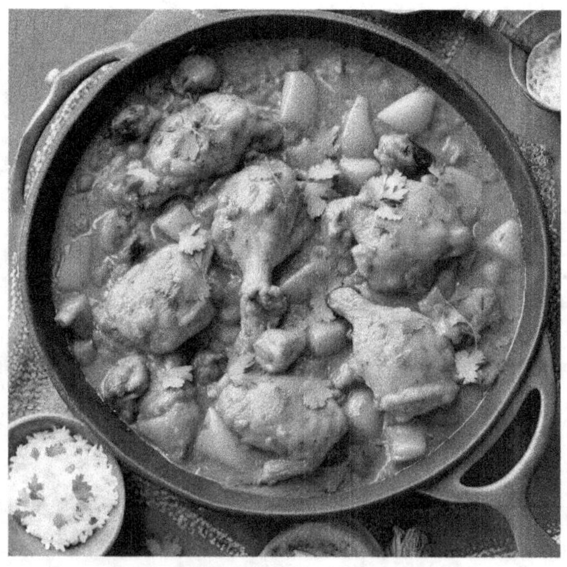

## 16. Chicken and Broccoli Alfredo

**Ingredients:**

- 1 lb boneless, skinless chicken breasts, sliced
- 2 tbsp olive oil
- 3 garlic cloves, minced
- 1 cup almond milk (or any dairy-free milk)
- 1/2 cup chicken broth (low sodium)
- 1/4 cup nutritional yeast
- 1 tbsp arrowroot powder (or cornstarch)
- 4 cups broccoli florets, steamed
- 1/4 cup fresh parsley, chopped

**Instructions:**

1. Heat olive oil in a large skillet over medium heat.
2. Add the sliced chicken and cook until browned, about 7-8 minutes. Remove from skillet and set aside.
3. In the same skillet, add minced garlic and cook for 1-2 minutes until fragrant.
4. In a small bowl, whisk together almond milk, chicken broth, nutritional yeast, and arrowroot powder.
5. Pour the mixture into the skillet, stirring constantly until the sauce thickens, about 5 minutes.
6. Add the cooked chicken and steamed broccoli to the skillet, stirring to combine.
7. Garnish with fresh parsley and serve immediately.

**Nutrition Info (per serving):**

- Calories: 300
- Protein: 28g
- Carbohydrates: 10g
- Fat: 16g
- Fiber: 4g
- Sugar: 3g

**Serves:**

4

**Cooking Time:**

30 minutes

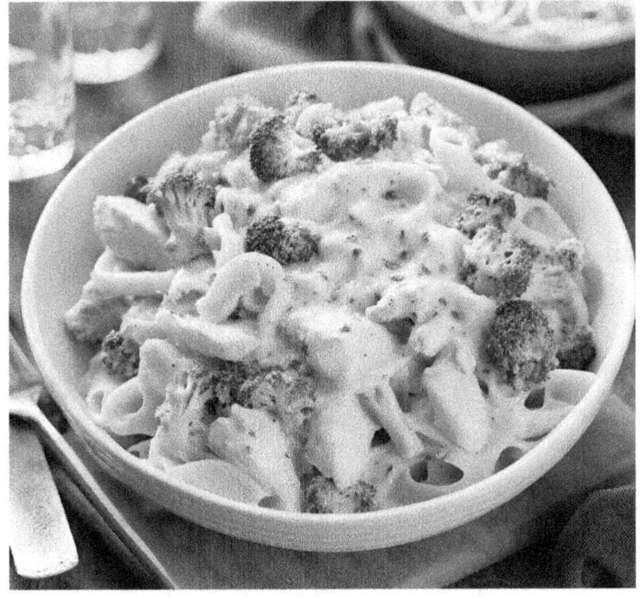

## 17. Roasted Turkey Breast with Rosemary and Sage

**Ingredients:**

- 1 turkey breast (about 2 lbs)
- 3 tbsp olive oil
- 2 garlic cloves, minced
- 1 tbsp fresh rosemary, chopped
- 1 tbsp fresh sage, chopped
- 1 lemon, juiced and zested
- 1/4 cup chicken broth (low sodium)

**Instructions:**

1. Preheat oven to 375°F (190°C).
2. In a small bowl, mix olive oil, minced garlic, rosemary, sage, lemon juice, and lemon zest.
3. Rub the mixture all over the turkey breast.
4. Place the turkey breast in a roasting pan and pour the chicken broth into the pan.
5. Roast for 1 hour and 15 minutes, or until the internal temperature reaches 165°F (74°C).
6. Let the turkey rest for 10 minutes before slicing.
7. Serve with the pan juices.

**Nutrition Info (per serving):**

- Calories: 320
- Protein: 32g
- Carbohydrates: 2g
- Fat: 20g
- Fiber: 1g
- Sugar: 0g

**Serves:**

4

**Cooking Time:**

1 hour 25 minutes

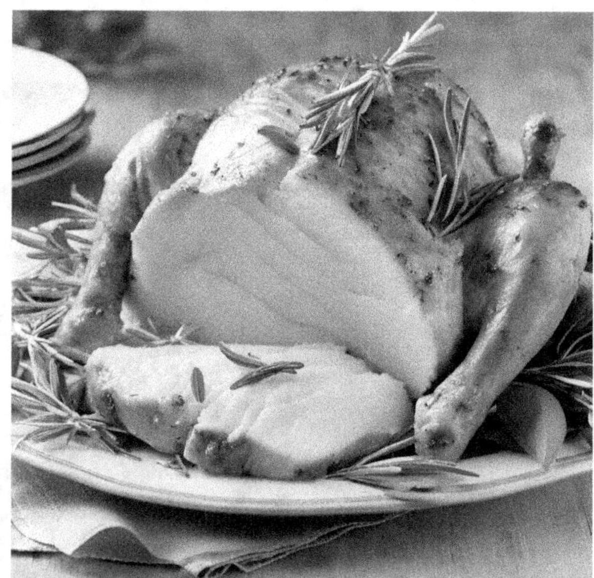

## 18. Chicken Paillard with Rocket Salad

**Ingredients:**

- 4 boneless, skinless chicken breasts
- 3 tbsp olive oil
- 1 lemon, juiced and zested
- 2 garlic cloves, minced
- 4 cups rocket (arugula)
- 1/2 cup cherry tomatoes, halved
- 1/4 cup shaved Parmesan cheese
- 1 tbsp balsamic vinegar

**Instructions:**

1. Pound the chicken breasts to about 1/4-inch thickness.
2. In a small bowl, mix 2 tbsp olive oil, lemon juice, lemon zest, and minced garlic.
3. Brush the chicken breasts with the olive oil mixture.
4. Heat the remaining olive oil in a large skillet over medium-high heat.
5. Cook the chicken for 2-3 minutes per side, until golden brown and cooked through.
6. In a large bowl, toss the rocket, cherry tomatoes, and Parmesan cheese with balsamic vinegar.
7. Serve the chicken paillard topped with the rocket salad.

**Nutrition Info (per serving):**

- Calories: 300
- Protein: 30g
- Carbohydrates: 6g
- Fat: 18g
- Fiber: 2g
- Sugar: 2g

**Serves:**

4

**Cooking Time:**

20 minutes

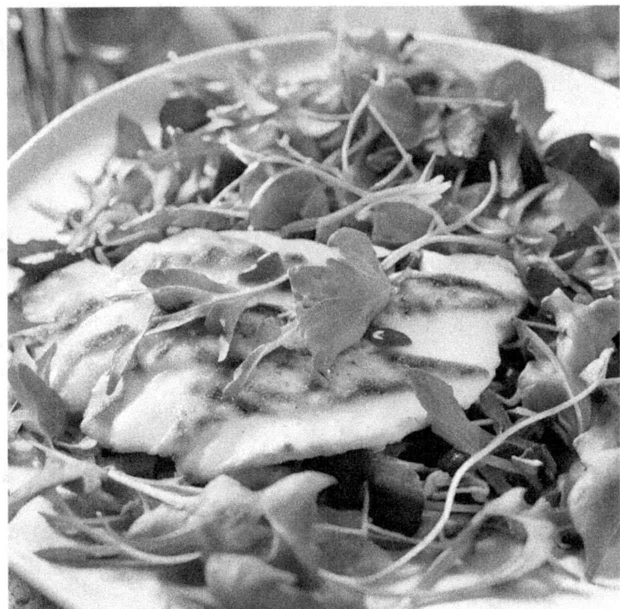

**19. Asian Turkey Lettuce Cups**

**Ingredients:**

- 1 lb ground turkey
- 2 tbsp olive oil
- 1 onion, finely chopped
- 2 garlic cloves, minced
- 1 tbsp ginger, minced
- 2 tbsp soy sauce (low sodium)
- 1 tbsp hoisin sauce
- 1 tbsp rice vinegar
- 1 cup water chestnuts, chopped
- 1/4 cup fresh cilantro, chopped
- 12 large lettuce leaves

**Instructions:**

1. Heat olive oil in a large skillet over medium heat.
2. Add the onion, garlic, and ginger, cooking until softened, about 5 minutes.
3. Add the ground turkey, cooking until browned, about 7-8 minutes.
4. Stir in the soy sauce, hoisin sauce, and rice vinegar, cooking for another 2 minutes.
5. Add the chopped water chestnuts and cilantro, stirring to combine.
6. Serve the turkey mixture in lettuce leaves.

**Nutrition Info (per serving, 3 cups):**

- Calories: 200
- Protein: 20g
- Carbohydrates: 10g
- Fat: 10g
- Fiber: 2g
- Sugar: 3g

**Serves:**

4

**Cooking Time:**

20 minutes

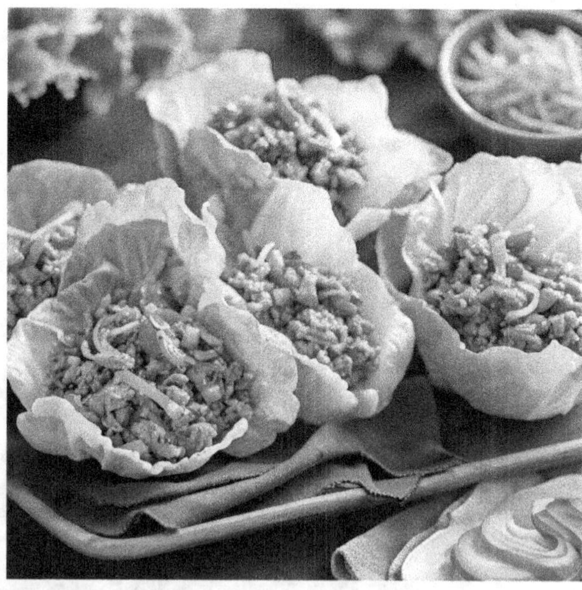

## 20. Chicken Vegetable Pot Pie

**Ingredients:**

- 1 lb boneless, skinless chicken breasts, diced
- 2 tbsp olive oil
- 1 onion, chopped
- 2 garlic cloves, minced
- 2 carrots, diced
- 2 celery stalks, diced
- 1 cup frozen peas
- 1 cup chicken broth (low sodium)
- 1 cup almond milk (or any dairy-free milk)
- 1/4 cup whole wheat flour
- 1 tsp dried thyme
- 1 sheet puff pastry (dairy-free if preferred)

**Instructions:**

1. Preheat oven to 375°F (190°C).
2. Heat olive oil in a large skillet over medium heat.
3. Add the onion, garlic, carrots, and celery, cooking until softened, about 5 minutes.
4. Add the diced chicken and cook until browned, about 7-8 minutes.
5. Stir in the whole wheat flour, cooking for 1-2 minutes.
6. Add the chicken broth, almond milk, frozen peas, and dried thyme, cooking until the mixture thickens, about 5 minutes.
7. Transfer the mixture to a baking dish and cover with the puff pastry sheet.
8. Bake for 20-25 minutes, or until the puff pastry is golden brown.
9. Serve hot.

**Nutrition Info (per serving):**

- Calories: 350
- Protein: 25g
- Carbohydrates: 30g
- Fat: 16g
- Fiber: 5g
- Sugar: 4g

**Serves:**

6

**Cooking Time:**

45 minutes

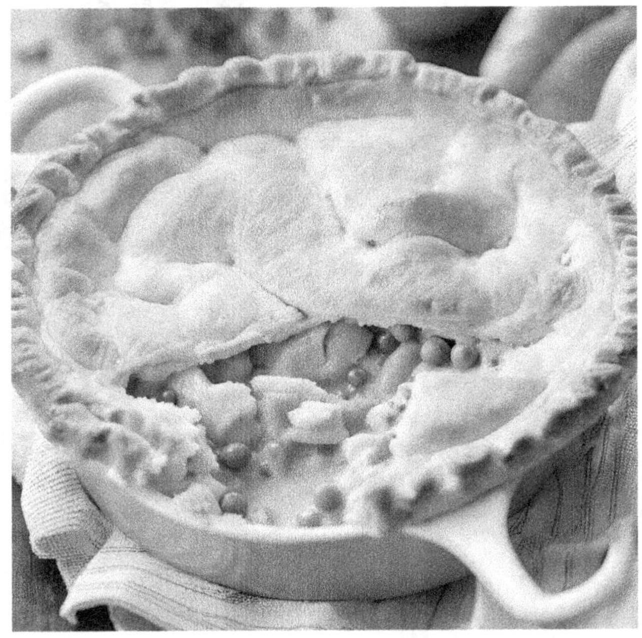

## 21. Baked Lemon Herb Chicken

**Ingredients:**

- 4 boneless, skinless chicken breasts
- 3 tbsp olive oil
- 1 lemon, juiced and zested
- 2 garlic cloves, minced
- 1 tbsp dried oregano
- 1 tbsp dried basil

**Instructions:**

1. Preheat oven to 375°F (190°C).
2. In a small bowl, mix olive oil, lemon juice, lemon zest, minced garlic, dried oregano, and dried basil.
3. Brush the mixture over the chicken breasts.
4. Place the chicken breasts in a baking dish.
5. Bake for 25-30 minutes, or until the chicken is cooked through.
6. Serve immediately.

**Nutrition Info (per serving):**

- Calories: 280
- Protein: 30g
- Carbohydrates: 2g
- Fat: 16g
- Fiber: 1g
- Sugar: 0g

**Serves:**

4

**Cooking Time:**

30 minutes

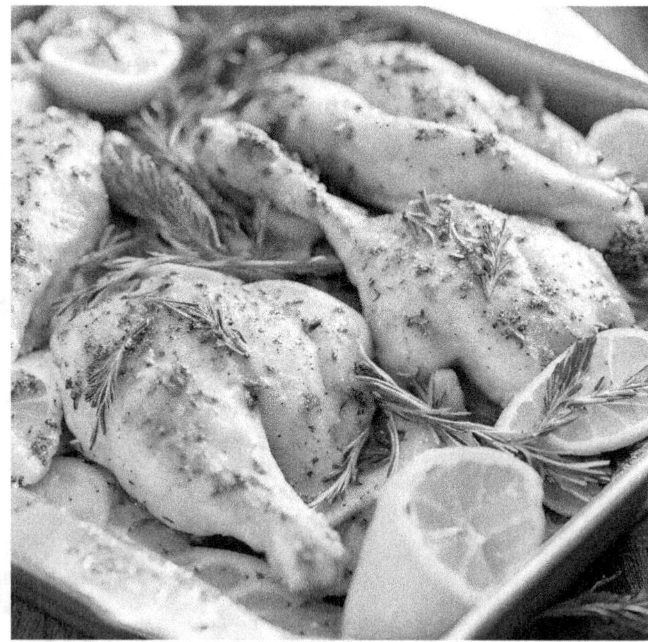

## 22. Chicken and Quinoa Salad

**Ingredients:**

- 1 lb boneless, skinless chicken breasts, cooked and diced
- 1 cup quinoa, cooked
- 1 cup cherry tomatoes, halved
- 1 cucumber, diced
- 1/4 cup red onion, finely chopped
- 1/4 cup feta cheese, crumbled
- 3 tbsp olive oil
- 1 lemon, juiced
- 1 tbsp fresh parsley, chopped

**Instructions:**

1. In a large bowl, combine the cooked chicken, cooked quinoa, cherry tomatoes, cucumber, red onion, and feta cheese.
2. In a small bowl, whisk together olive oil, lemon juice, and fresh parsley.
3. Pour the dressing over the salad and toss to combine.
4. Serve immediately or chill until ready to serve.

**Nutrition Info (per serving):**

- Calories: 320
- Protein: 28g
- Carbohydrates: 20g
- Fat: 14g
- Fiber: 4g
- Sugar: 4g

**Serves:**

4

**Cooking Time:**

20 minutes

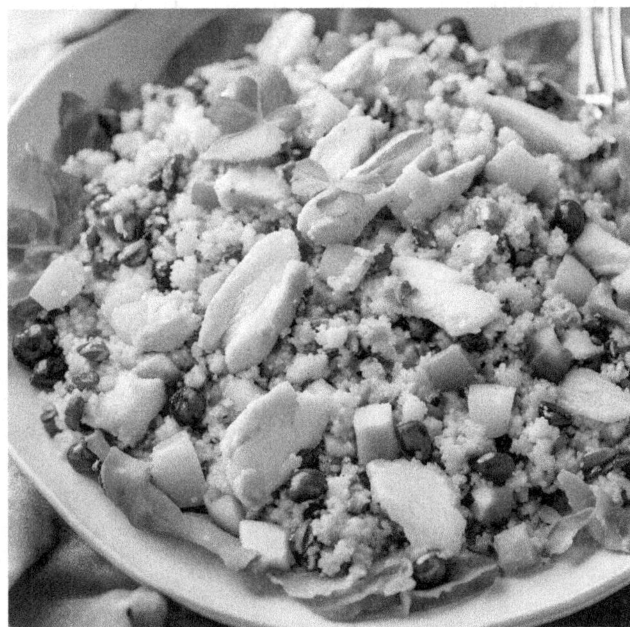

### 23. Chicken Ratatouille

**Ingredients:**

- 1 lb boneless, skinless chicken breasts, diced
- 3 tbsp olive oil
- 1 onion, chopped
- 2 garlic cloves, minced
- 1 eggplant, diced
- 1 zucchini, diced
- 1 red bell pepper, diced
- 1 can (14 oz) diced tomatoes
- 1 tsp dried basil
- 1 tsp dried oregano
- 1/4 tsp black pepper

**Instructions:**

1. Heat 2 tbsp olive oil in a large skillet over medium heat.
2. Add the onion and garlic, cooking until softened, about 5 minutes.
3. Add the diced chicken, cooking until browned, about 7-8 minutes.
4. Remove the chicken from the skillet and set aside.
5. Add the remaining olive oil to the skillet, then add the diced eggplant, zucchini, and red bell pepper. Cook for about 5-7 minutes until the vegetables are tender.
6. Stir in the diced tomatoes, dried basil, dried oregano, and black pepper.
7. Return the chicken to the skillet and stir to combine.
8. Simmer for 15-20 minutes until the flavors are well combined and the chicken is cooked through.
9. Serve hot.

**Nutrition Info (per serving):**

- Calories: 300
- Protein: 26g
- Carbohydrates: 16g
- Fat: 16g
- Fiber: 5g
- Sugar: 9g

**Serves:**

4

**Cooking Time:**

35 minutes

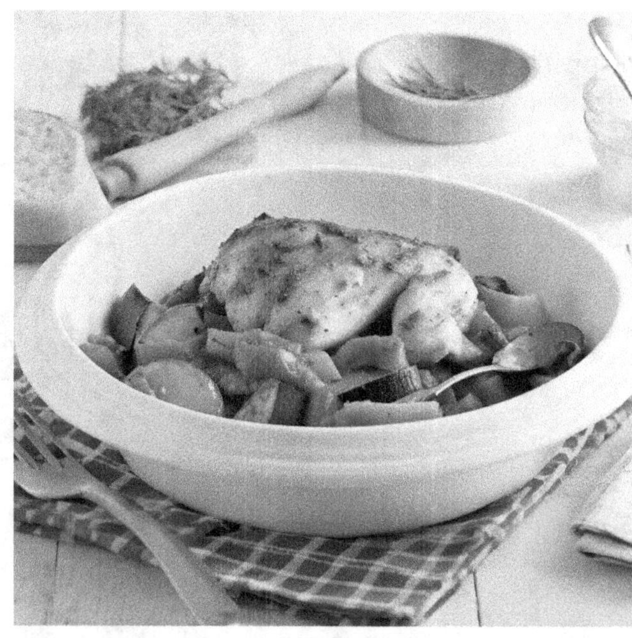

## 24. Herb-Roasted Chicken

**Ingredients:**

- 1 whole chicken (about 4 lbs)
- 3 tbsp olive oil
- 4 garlic cloves, minced
- 1 tbsp fresh rosemary, chopped
- 1 tbsp fresh thyme, chopped
- 1 lemon, halved
- 1 cup chicken broth (low sodium)

**Instructions:**

1. Preheat oven to 375°F (190°C).
2. In a small bowl, mix olive oil, minced garlic, rosemary, and thyme.
3. Rub the herb mixture all over the chicken.
4. Place the lemon halves inside the chicken cavity.
5. Place the chicken in a roasting pan and pour the chicken broth into the pan.
6. Roast for 1 hour and 30 minutes, or until the internal temperature reaches 165°F (74°C).
7. Let the chicken rest for 10 minutes before carving.
8. Serve with the pan juices.

**Nutrition Info (per serving):**

- Calories: 450
- Protein: 35g
- Carbohydrates: 2g
- Fat: 32g
- Fiber: 1g
- Sugar: 0g

**Serves:**

6

**Cooking Time:**

1 hour 40 minutes

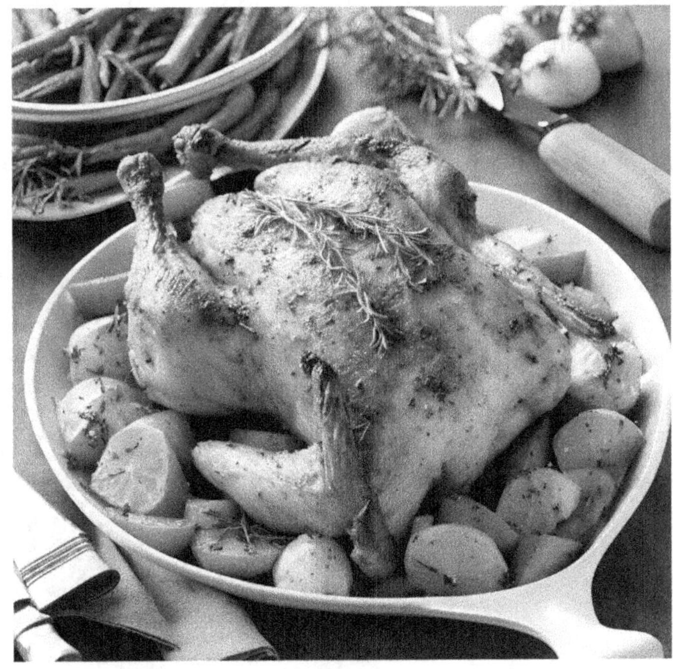

# Soups and Stew

**1. Carrot Ginger Soup**

**Ingredients:**

- 1 lb carrots, peeled and chopped
- 1 onion, chopped
- 3 garlic cloves, minced
- 1 tbsp ginger, minced
- 2 tbsp olive oil
- 4 cups vegetable broth (low sodium)
- 1 cup coconut milk
- 1 tbsp lemon juice
- 1/4 tsp cumin
- 1/4 tsp turmeric
- 1/4 cup fresh cilantro, chopped (optional for garnish)

**Instructions:**

1. Heat olive oil in a large pot over medium heat.
2. Add the onion, garlic, and ginger, cooking until softened, about 5 minutes.
3. Add the chopped carrots, cumin, and turmeric, stirring to combine.
4. Pour in the vegetable broth and bring to a boil.
5. Reduce heat and simmer for 20-25 minutes, or until the carrots are tender.
6. Use an immersion blender or transfer the soup to a blender to puree until smooth.
7. Stir in the coconut milk and lemon juice, heating through.
8. Garnish with fresh cilantro if desired, and serve hot.

**Nutrition Info (per serving):**

- Calories: 180
- Protein: 2g
- Carbohydrates: 22g
- Fat: 10g
- Fiber: 5g
- Sugar: 9g

**Serves:**

4

**Cooking Time:**

35 minutes

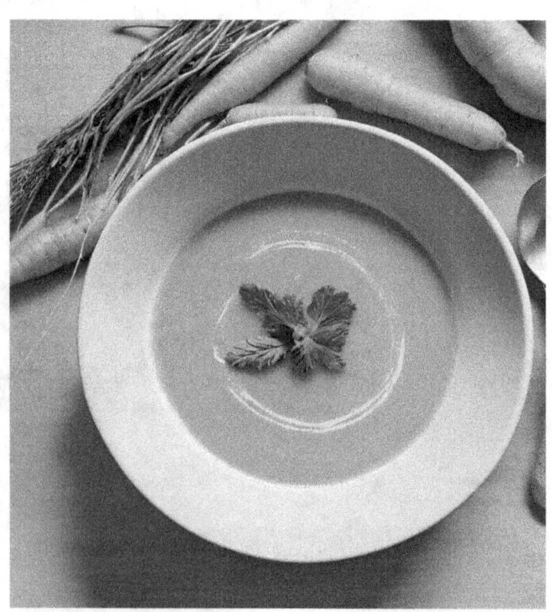

## 2. Turmeric Chicken Soup

**Ingredients:**

- 1 lb boneless, skinless chicken breasts, diced
- 2 tbsp olive oil
- 1 onion, chopped
- 3 garlic cloves, minced
- 1 tbsp ginger, minced
- 1 tsp ground turmeric
- 4 cups chicken broth (low sodium)
- 2 carrots, sliced
- 2 celery stalks, sliced
- 1 cup coconut milk
- 1 tbsp lemon juice
- 1/4 cup fresh cilantro, chopped (optional for garnish)

**Instructions:**

1. Heat olive oil in a large pot over medium heat.
2. Add the onion, garlic, and ginger, cooking until softened, about 5 minutes.
3. Add the diced chicken and cook until browned, about 7-8 minutes.
4. Stir in the ground turmeric and cook for another 2 minutes.
5. Add the chicken broth, carrots, and celery, bringing to a boil.
6. Reduce heat and simmer for 20-25 minutes, or until the vegetables are tender and the chicken is cooked through.
7. Stir in the coconut milk and lemon juice, heating through.
8. Garnish with fresh cilantro if desired, and serve hot.

**Nutrition Info (per serving):**

- Calories: 220
- Protein: 22g
- Carbohydrates: 10g
- Fat: 12g
- Fiber: 3g
- Sugar: 5g

**Serves:**

4

**Cooking Time:**

35 minutes

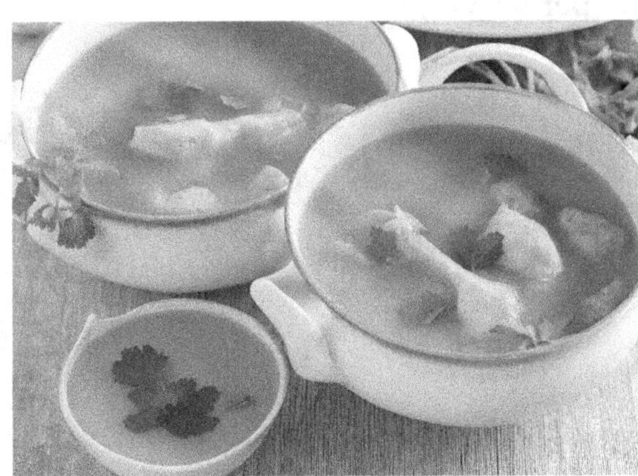

### 3. Vegetable Minestrone

**Ingredients:**

- 2 tbsp olive oil
- 1 onion, chopped
- 3 garlic cloves, minced
- 2 carrots, diced
- 2 celery stalks, diced
- 1 zucchini, diced
- 1 can (14 oz) diced tomatoes
- 4 cups vegetable broth (low sodium)
- 1 cup cooked cannellini beans
- 1 cup spinach, chopped
- 1 tsp dried basil
- 1 tsp dried oregano
- 1/4 cup fresh parsley, chopped (optional for garnish)

**Instructions:**

1. Heat olive oil in a large pot over medium heat.
2. Add the onion and garlic, cooking until softened, about 5 minutes.
3. Stir in the carrots, celery, and zucchini, cooking for another 5 minutes.
4. Add the diced tomatoes, vegetable broth, cooked cannellini beans, dried basil, and dried oregano.
5. Bring to a boil, then reduce heat and simmer for 20-25 minutes, or until the vegetables are tender.
6. Stir in the chopped spinach and cook for another 5 minutes until wilted.
7. Garnish with fresh parsley if desired, and serve hot.

**Nutrition Info (per serving):**

- Calories: 180
- Protein: 6g
- Carbohydrates: 26g
- Fat: 6g
- Fiber: 6g
- Sugar: 9g

**Serves:**

4

**Cooking Time:**

35 minutes

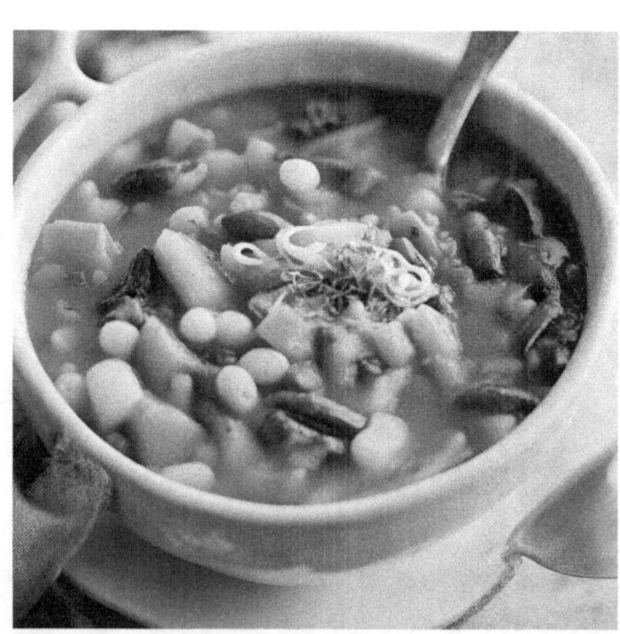

## 4. Miso Soup with Tofu and Seaweed

**Ingredients:**

- 4 cups water
- 1/4 cup miso paste
- 1 cup tofu, cubed
- 1/4 cup dried seaweed (wakame)
- 2 green onions, sliced
- 1 tbsp soy sauce (low sodium)
- 1 tbsp sesame oil

**Instructions:**

1. In a medium pot, bring the water to a simmer over medium heat.
2. Add the miso paste, stirring until dissolved.
3. Add the cubed tofu and dried seaweed, cooking for 5-7 minutes until the seaweed is rehydrated and the tofu is heated through.
4. Stir in the soy sauce and sesame oil.
5. Garnish with sliced green onions and serve hot.

**Nutrition Info (per serving):**

- Calories: 120
- Protein: 6g
- Carbohydrates: 8g
- Fat: 8g
- Fiber: 2g
- Sugar: 2g

**Serves:**

4

**Cooking Time:**

15 minutes

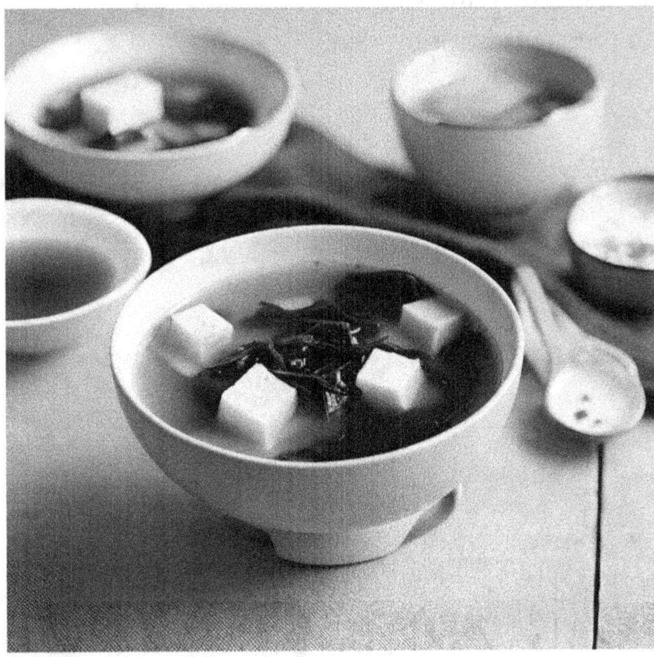

**5. Thai Coconut Shrimp Soup**
**Ingredients:**
- 1 lb shrimp, peeled and deveined
- 2 tbsp olive oil
- 1 onion, chopped
- 3 garlic cloves, minced
- 1 tbsp ginger, minced
- 2 cups coconut milk
- 3 cups chicken broth (low sodium)
- 1 red bell pepper, sliced
- 1 cup mushrooms, sliced
- 1 tbsp fish sauce
- 1 tbsp lime juice
- 1/4 cup fresh cilantro, chopped (optional for garnish)

**Instructions:**
1. Heat olive oil in a large pot over medium heat.
2. Add the onion, garlic, and ginger, cooking until softened, about 5 minutes.
3. Stir in the coconut milk, chicken broth, red bell pepper, mushrooms, and fish sauce. Bring to a boil.
4. Reduce heat and simmer for 10 minutes.
5. Add the shrimp and cook until pink and opaque, about 3-4 minutes.
6. Stir in the lime juice.
7. Garnish with fresh cilantro if desired, and serve hot.

**Nutrition Info (per serving):**
- Calories: 320
- Protein: 22g
- Carbohydrates: 12g
- Fat: 22g
- Fiber: 3g
- Sugar: 5g

**Serves:**
4
**Cooking Time:**
30 minutes

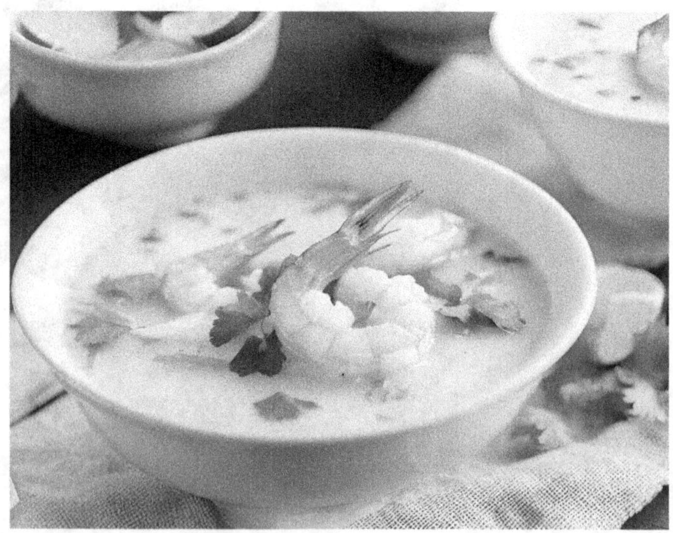

## 6. Beetroot and Ginger Soup

**Ingredients:**

- 1 lb beetroots, peeled and chopped
- 1 onion, chopped
- 2 garlic cloves, minced
- 1 tbsp ginger, minced
- 2 tbsp olive oil
- 4 cups vegetable broth (low sodium)
- 1 tbsp lemon juice
- 1/4 cup coconut milk (optional for garnish)

**Instructions:**

1. Heat olive oil in a large pot over medium heat.
2. Add the onion, garlic, and ginger, cooking until softened, about 5 minutes.
3. Add the chopped beetroots and vegetable broth. Bring to a boil.
4. Reduce heat and simmer for 25-30 minutes, or until the beetroots are tender.
5. Use an immersion blender or transfer the soup to a blender to puree until smooth.
6. Stir in the lemon juice.
7. Garnish with a drizzle of coconut milk if desired, and serve hot.

**Nutrition Info (per serving):**

- Calories: 160
- Protein: 2g
- Carbohydrates: 20g
- Fat: 8g
- Fiber: 5g
- Sugar: 14g

**Serves:**

4

**Cooking Time:**

40 minutes

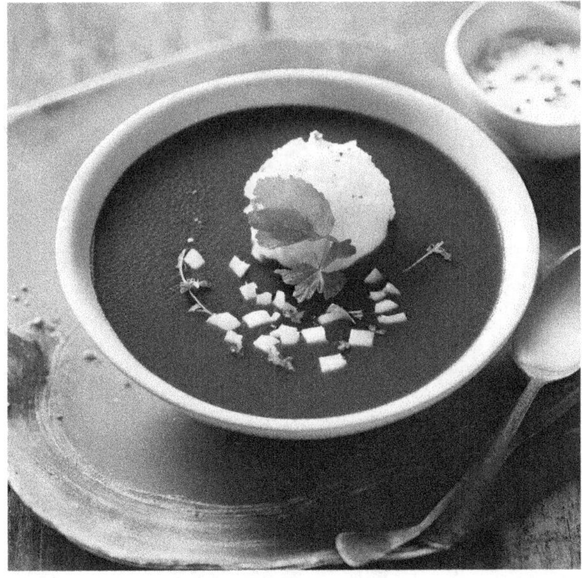

## 7. Broccoli Almond Soup

**Ingredients:**

- 1 lb broccoli florets
- 1 onion, chopped
- 3 garlic cloves, minced
- 2 tbsp olive oil
- 1/4 cup raw almonds
- 4 cups vegetable broth (low sodium)
- 1 cup almond milk
- 1 tbsp lemon juice

**Instructions:**

1. Heat olive oil in a large pot over medium heat.
2. Add the onion and garlic, cooking until softened, about 5 minutes.
3. Add the broccoli florets and raw almonds, stirring to combine.
4. Pour in the vegetable broth and bring to a boil.
5. Reduce heat and simmer for 20 minutes, or until the broccoli is tender.
6. Use an immersion blender or transfer the soup to a blender to puree until smooth.
7. Stir in the almond milk and lemon juice, heating through.
8. Serve hot.

**Nutrition Info (per serving):**

- Calories: 180
- Protein: 6g
- Carbohydrates: 14g
- Fat: 12g
- Fiber: 5g
- Sugar: 5g

**Serves:**

4

**Cooking Time:**

30 minutes

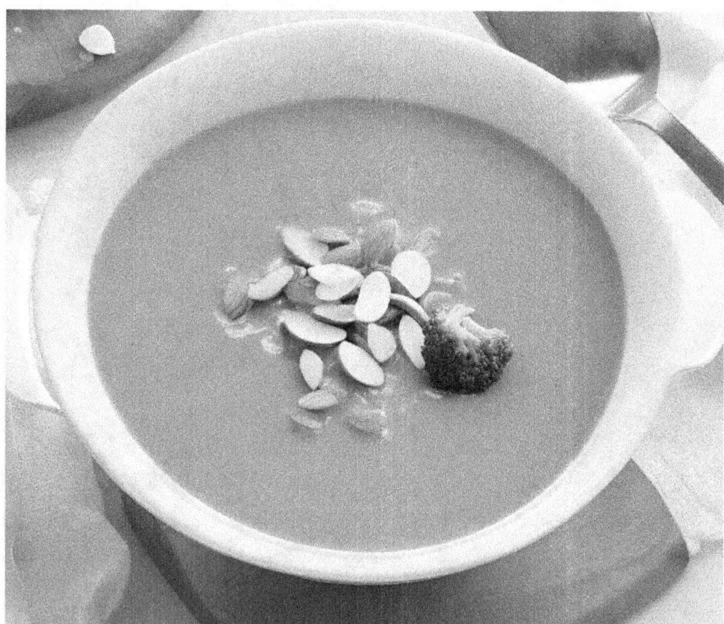

## 8. Sweet Potato and Black Bean Chili

**Ingredients:**

- 2 tbsp olive oil
- 1 onion, chopped
- 3 garlic cloves, minced
- 1 lb sweet potatoes, peeled and diced
- 1 red bell pepper, chopped
- 1 can (14 oz) black beans, drained and rinsed
- 1 can (14 oz) diced tomatoes
- 2 cups vegetable broth (low sodium)
- 1 tbsp chili powder
- 1 tsp cumin
- 1/4 cup fresh cilantro, chopped (optional for garnish)

**Instructions:**

1. Heat olive oil in a large pot over medium heat.
2. Add the onion and garlic, cooking until softened, about 5 minutes.
3. Add the sweet potatoes, red bell pepper, black beans, diced tomatoes, vegetable broth, chili powder, and cumin. Stir to combine.
4. Bring to a boil, then reduce heat and simmer for 25-30 minutes, or until the sweet potatoes are tender.
5. Garnish with fresh cilantro if desired, and serve hot.

**Nutrition Info (per serving):**

- Calories: 240
- Protein: 7g
- Carbohydrates: 40g
- Fat: 6g
- Fiber: 10g
- Sugar: 10g

**Serves:**

4

**Cooking Time:**

40 minutes

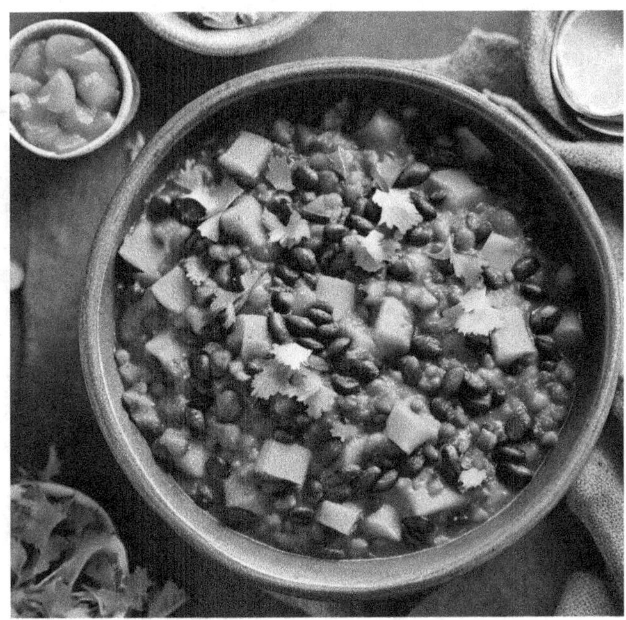

**9. Zucchini Soup**

**Ingredients:**

- 2 tbsp olive oil
- 1 onion, chopped
- 3 garlic cloves, minced
- 4 zucchini, chopped
- 4 cups vegetable broth (low sodium)
- 1/2 cup coconut milk
- 1 tbsp lemon juice
- 1/4 cup fresh basil, chopped (optional for garnish)

**Instructions:**

1. Heat olive oil in a large pot over medium heat.
2. Add the onion and garlic, cooking until softened, about 5 minutes.
3. Add the chopped zucchini and vegetable broth. Bring to a boil.
4. Reduce heat and simmer for 20 minutes, or until the zucchini is tender.
5. Use an immersion blender or transfer the soup to a blender to puree until smooth.
6. Stir in the coconut milk and lemon juice, heating through.
7. Garnish with fresh basil if desired, and serve hot.

**Nutrition Info (per serving):**

- Calories: 150
- Protein: 3g
- Carbohydrates: 10g
- Fat: 10g
- Fiber: 2g
- Sugar: 5g

**Serves:**

4

**Cooking Time:**

30 minutes

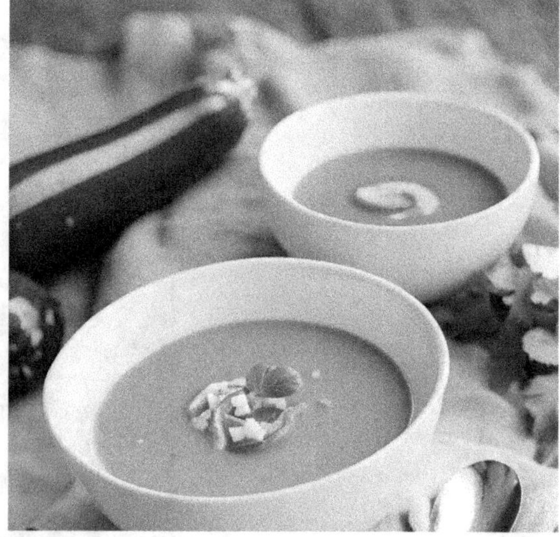

## 10. Kale and Potato Soup

**Ingredients:**

- 2 tbsp olive oil
- 1 onion, chopped
- 3 garlic cloves, minced
- 4 cups kale, chopped
- 2 potatoes, peeled and diced
- 4 cups vegetable broth (low sodium)
- 1/2 cup coconut milk
- 1/4 tsp thyme
- 1 tbsp apple cider vinegar

**Instructions:**

1. Heat olive oil in a large pot over medium heat.
2. Add the onion and garlic, cooking until softened, about 5 minutes.
3. Add the chopped kale and diced potatoes, stirring to combine.
4. Pour in the vegetable broth and bring to a boil.
5. Reduce heat and simmer for 20-25 minutes, or until the potatoes are tender.
6. Use an immersion blender or transfer half of the soup to a blender to puree, then return to the pot.
7. Stir in the coconut milk, thyme, and apple cider vinegar, heating through.
8. Serve hot.

**Nutrition Info (per serving):**

- Calories: 180
- Protein: 4g
- Carbohydrates: 20g
- Fat: 10g
- Fiber: 4g
- Sugar: 5g

**Serves:**

4

**Cooking Time:**

35 minutes

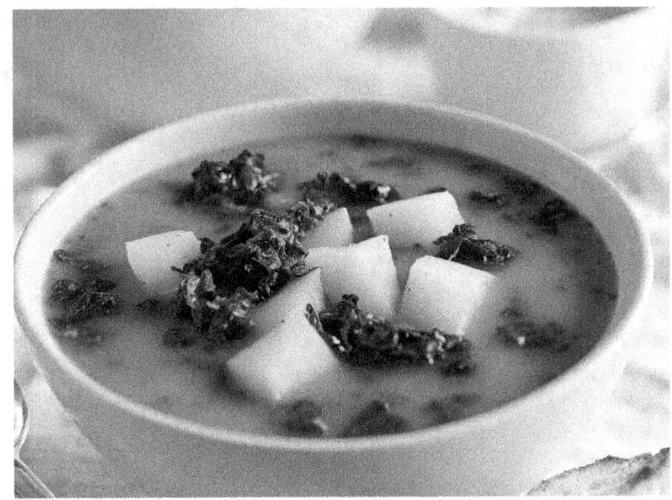

## 11. Bok Choy and Mushroom Soup

**Ingredients:**

- 2 tbsp olive oil
- 1 onion, chopped
- 3 garlic cloves, minced
- 1 inch ginger, minced
- 4 cups vegetable broth (low sodium)
- 2 cups mushrooms, sliced
- 4 cups bok choy, chopped
- 1 tbsp soy sauce (low sodium)
- 1 tbsp sesame oil
- 1/4 cup green onions, sliced (optional for garnish)

**Instructions:**

1. Heat olive oil in a large pot over medium heat.
2. Add the onion, garlic, and ginger, cooking until softened, about 5 minutes.
3. Add the vegetable broth and bring to a boil.
4. Stir in the sliced mushrooms and chopped bok choy, cooking for 10 minutes until tender.
5. Add the soy sauce and sesame oil, stirring to combine.
6. Garnish with sliced green onions if desired, and serve hot.

**Nutrition Info (per serving):**

- Calories: 140
- Protein: 4g
- Carbohydrates: 10g
- Fat: 10g
- Fiber: 2g
- Sugar: 4g

**Serves:**

4

**Cooking Time:**

25 minutes

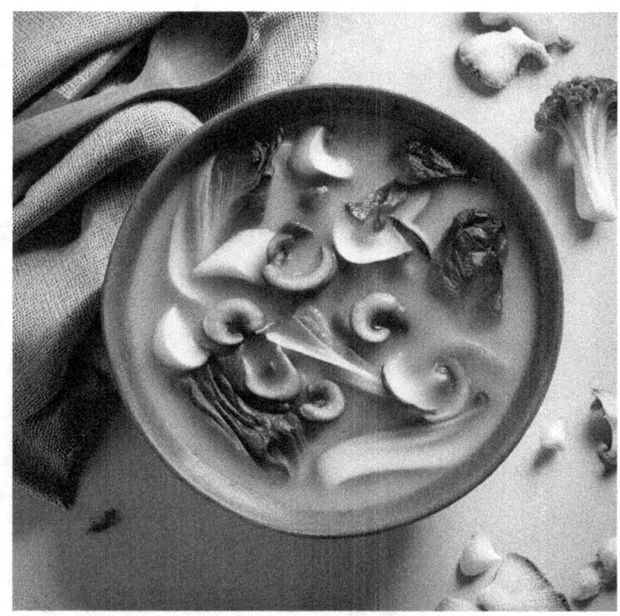

## 12. Spicy Tomato and Lentil Soup

**Ingredients:**

- 2 tbsp olive oil
- 1 onion, chopped
- 3 garlic cloves, minced
- 1 tbsp ginger, minced
- 1 tsp ground cumin
- 1 tsp ground coriander
- 1/2 tsp cayenne pepper
- 1 cup red lentils, rinsed
- 1 can (14 oz) diced tomatoes
- 4 cups vegetable broth (low sodium)
- 1 tbsp lemon juice
- 1/4 cup fresh cilantro, chopped (optional for garnish)

**Instructions:**

1. Heat olive oil in a large pot over medium heat.
2. Add the onion, garlic, and ginger, cooking until softened, about 5 minutes.
3. Stir in the ground cumin, ground coriander, and cayenne pepper, cooking for another 2 minutes.
4. Add the red lentils, diced tomatoes, and vegetable broth. Bring to a boil.
5. Reduce heat and simmer for 20-25 minutes, or until the lentils are tender.
6. Stir in the lemon juice.
7. Garnish with fresh cilantro if desired, and serve hot.

**Nutrition Info (per serving):**

- Calories: 220
- Protein: 10g
- Carbohydrates: 30g
- Fat: 7g
- Fiber: 9g
- Sugar: 6g

**Serves:**

4

**Cooking Time:**

30 minutes

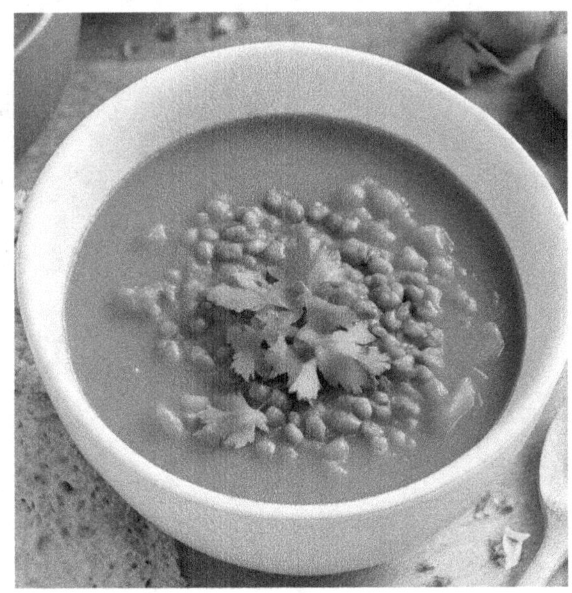

**13. Celery Soup**

**Ingredients:**

- 2 tbsp olive oil
- 1 onion, chopped
- 3 garlic cloves, minced
- 6 cups celery, chopped
- 4 cups vegetable broth (low sodium)
- 1 cup almond milk
- 1 tsp dried thyme
- 1 tbsp lemon juice

**Instructions:**

1. Heat olive oil in a large pot over medium heat.
2. Add the onion and garlic, cooking until softened, about 5 minutes.
3. Add the chopped celery and cook for another 5 minutes.
4. Pour in the vegetable broth and bring to a boil.
5. Reduce heat and simmer for 20-25 minutes, or until the celery is tender.
6. Use an immersion blender or transfer the soup to a blender to puree until smooth.
7. Stir in the almond milk, dried thyme, and lemon juice, heating through.
8. Serve hot.

**Nutrition Info (per serving):**

- Calories: 150
- Protein: 3g
- Carbohydrates: 12g
- Fat: 10g
- Fiber: 4g
- Sugar: 4g

**Serves:**

4

**Cooking Time:**

35 minutes

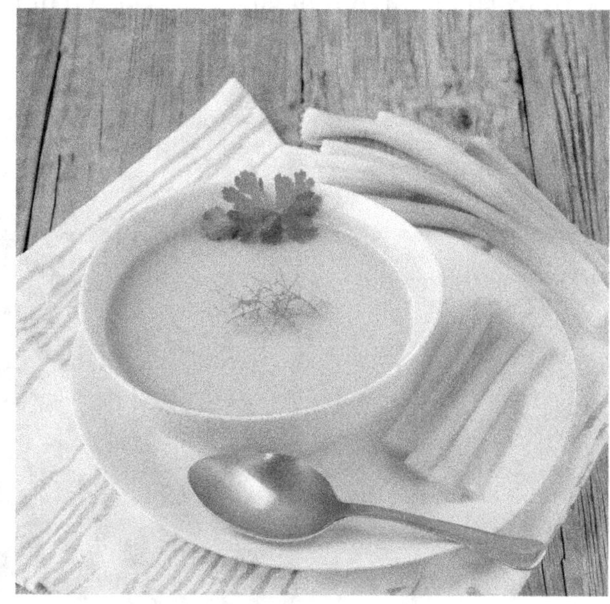

## 14. Split Pea Soup

**Ingredients:**

- 2 tbsp olive oil
- 1 onion, chopped
- 3 garlic cloves, minced
- 2 carrots, diced
- 2 celery stalks, diced
- 2 cups split peas, rinsed
- 6 cups vegetable broth (low sodium)
- 1 tsp dried thyme
- 1 bay leaf
- 1 tbsp apple cider vinegar

**Instructions:**

1. Heat olive oil in a large pot over medium heat.
2. Add the onion, garlic, carrots, and celery, cooking until softened, about 5 minutes.
3. Stir in the split peas, vegetable broth, dried thyme, and bay leaf. Bring to a boil.
4. Reduce heat and simmer for 45-50 minutes, or until the split peas are tender.
5. Remove the bay leaf and stir in the apple cider vinegar.
6. Serve hot.

**Nutrition Info (per serving):**

- Calories: 280
- Protein: 15g
- Carbohydrates: 45g
- Fat: 6g
- Fiber: 16g
- Sugar: 8g

**Serves:**

4

**Cooking Time:**

55 minutes

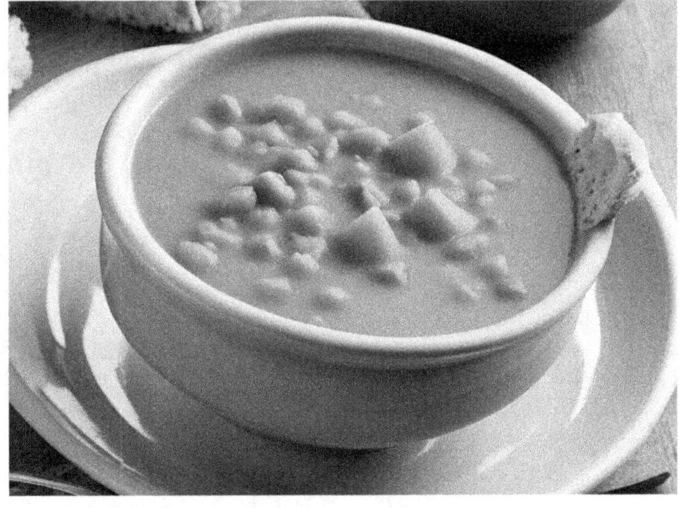

**15. Egg Drop Soup**

**Ingredients:**

- 4 cups chicken broth (low sodium)
- 1 tbsp soy sauce (low sodium)
- 1 tsp sesame oil
- 2 eggs, beaten
- 2 green onions, sliced
- 1/2 cup mushrooms, sliced (optional)

**Instructions:**

1. In a medium pot, bring the chicken broth, soy sauce, and sesame oil to a boil.
2. Reduce heat to a simmer and add the sliced mushrooms if using.
3. Slowly pour the beaten eggs into the pot, stirring gently to create ribbons of egg.
4. Cook for another 2 minutes until the eggs are set.
5. Garnish with sliced green onions and serve hot.

**Nutrition Info (per serving):**

- Calories: 90
- Protein: 6g
- Carbohydrates: 3g
- Fat: 6g
- Fiber: 1g
- Sugar: 1g

**Serves:**

4

**Cooking Time:**

15 minutes

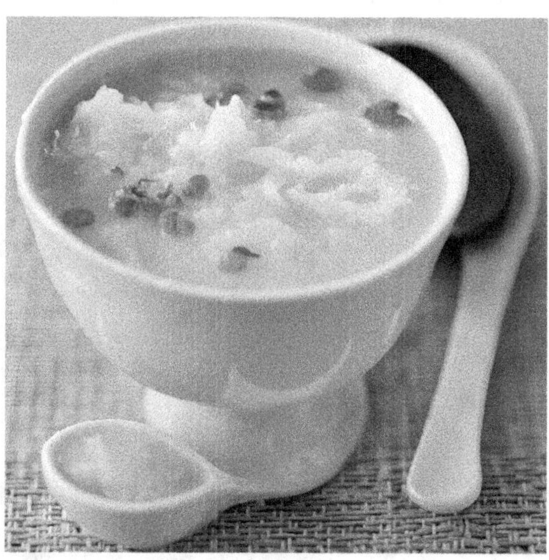

**16. Cabbage Soup**

**Ingredients:**

- 2 tbsp olive oil
- 1 onion, chopped
- 3 garlic cloves, minced
- 4 cups cabbage, chopped
- 2 carrots, sliced
- 2 celery stalks, sliced
- 1 can (14 oz) diced tomatoes
- 4 cups vegetable broth (low sodium)
- 1 tsp dried basil
- 1 tsp dried oregano
- 1 tbsp apple cider vinegar

**Instructions:**

1. Heat olive oil in a large pot over medium heat.
2. Add the onion and garlic, cooking until softened, about 5 minutes.
3. Add the chopped cabbage, carrots, and celery, stirring to combine.
4. Pour in the diced tomatoes, vegetable broth, dried basil, and dried oregano. Bring to a boil.
5. Reduce heat and simmer for 25-30 minutes, or until the vegetables are tender.
6. Stir in the apple cider vinegar.
7. Serve hot.

**Nutrition Info (per serving):**

- Calories: 120
- Protein: 3g
- Carbohydrates: 18g
- Fat: 5g
- Fiber: 6g
- Sugar: 9g

**Serves:**

4

**Cooking Time:**

35 minutes

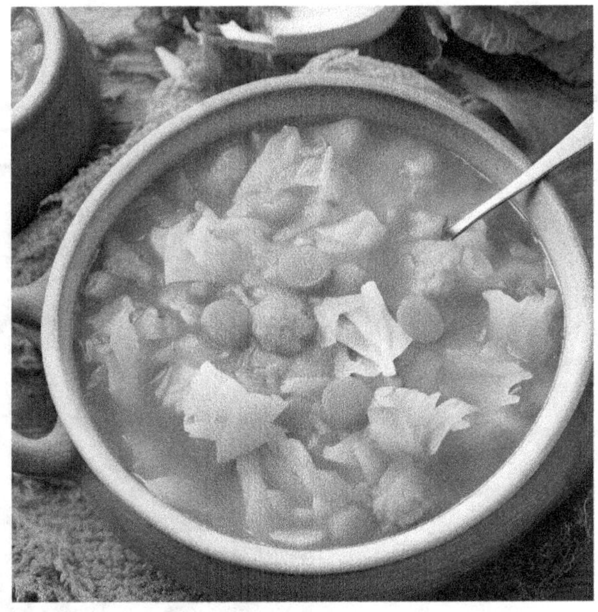

## 17. Moroccan Chickpea Stew

**Ingredients:**

- 2 tbsp olive oil
- 1 onion, chopped
- 3 garlic cloves, minced
- 1 tbsp ginger, minced
- 1 tsp ground cumin
- 1 tsp ground coriander
- 1/2 tsp ground cinnamon
- 1/4 tsp cayenne pepper
- 1 can (14 oz) diced tomatoes
- 2 cups vegetable broth (low sodium)
- 1 can (14 oz) chickpeas, drained and rinsed
- 1 sweet potato, peeled and diced
- 1/2 cup dried apricots, chopped
- 1/4 cup fresh cilantro, chopped (optional for garnish)

**Instructions:**

1. Heat olive oil in a large pot over medium heat.
2. Add the onion, garlic, and ginger, cooking until softened, about 5 minutes.
3. Stir in the ground cumin, ground coriander, ground cinnamon, and cayenne pepper, cooking for another 2 minutes until fragrant.
4. Add the diced tomatoes, vegetable broth, chickpeas, sweet potato, and dried apricots. Stir to combine.
5. Bring to a boil, then reduce heat and simmer for 25-30 minutes, or until the sweet potato is tender.
6. Garnish with fresh cilantro if desired, and serve hot.

**Nutrition Info (per serving):**

- Calories: 300
- Protein: 8g
- Carbohydrates: 50g
- Fat: 8g
- Fiber: 10g
- Sugar: 18g

**Serves:**

4

**Cooking Time:**

40 minutes

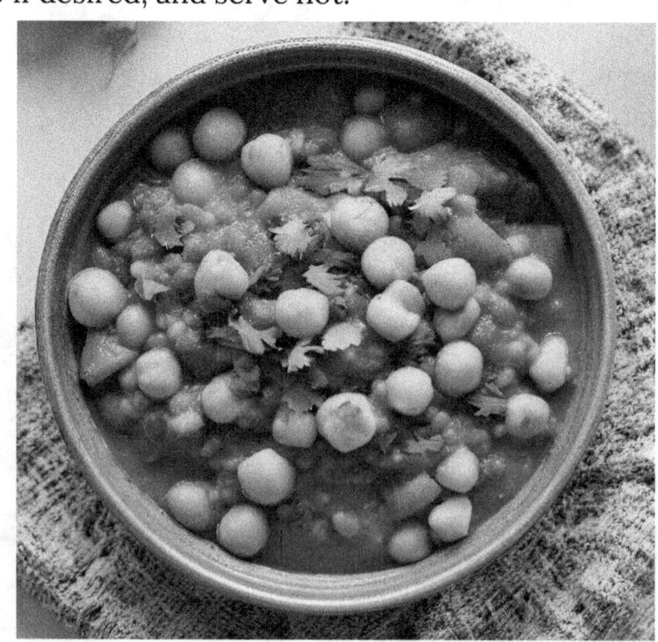

## 18. Mushroom and Tarragon Soup

**Ingredients:**

- 2 tbsp olive oil
- 1 onion, chopped
- 3 garlic cloves, minced
- 1 lb mushrooms, sliced
- 4 cups vegetable broth (low sodium)
- 1 cup almond milk
- 1 tbsp fresh tarragon, chopped
- 1 tbsp lemon juice

**Instructions:**

1. Heat olive oil in a large pot over medium heat.
2. Add the
3. Add the                                                           gin to brown, about 10
4. Pour in t
5. Reduce h
6. Stir in th                                                        ough.
7. Serve ho

**Nutrition In**

- Calories:
- Protein:
- Carbohy
- Fat: 10g
- Fiber: 3g
- Sugar: 5g

**Serves:**

4

**Cooking Tim**

30 minutes

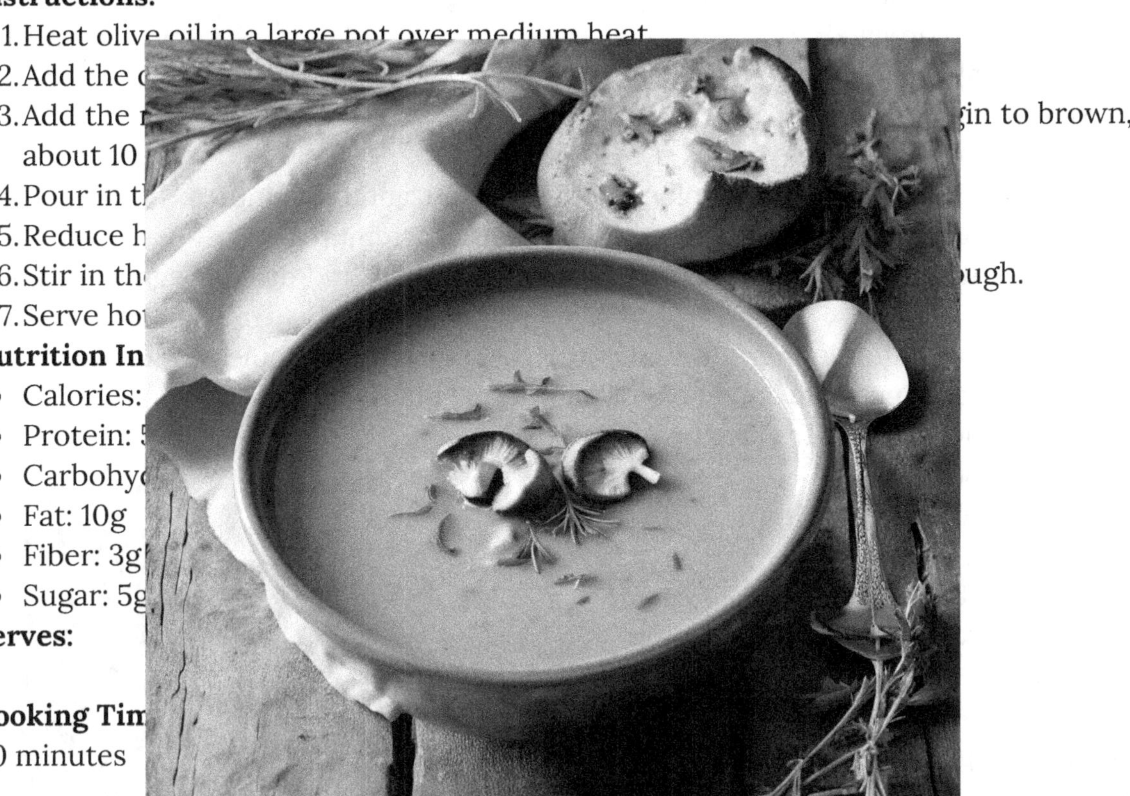

### 19. Italian White Bean and Kale Soup

**Ingredients:**

- 2 tbsp olive oil
- 1 onion, chopped
- 3 garlic cloves, minced
- 2 carrots, diced
- 2 celery stalks, diced
- 1 can (14 oz) white beans, drained and rinsed
- 4 cups vegetable broth (low sodium)
- 4 cups kale, chopped
- 1 tsp dried basil
- 1 tsp dried oregano
- 1 tbsp apple cider vinegar

**Instructions:**

1. Heat olive oil in a large pot over medium heat.
2. Add the onion and garlic, cooking until softened, about 5 minutes.
3. Add the carrots and celery, cooking for another 5 minutes.
4. Stir in the white beans, vegetable broth, dried basil, and dried oregano. Bring to a boil.
5. Reduce heat and simmer for 20 minutes, or until the vegetables are tender.
6. Add the chopped kale and cook for another 5 minutes until wilted.
7. Stir in the apple cider vinegar.
8. Serve hot.

**Nutrition Info (per serving):**

- Calories: 200
- Protein: 8g
- Carbohydrates: 30g
- Fat: 7g
- Fiber: 8g
- Sugar: 6g

**Serves:**

4

**Cooking Time:**

35 minutes

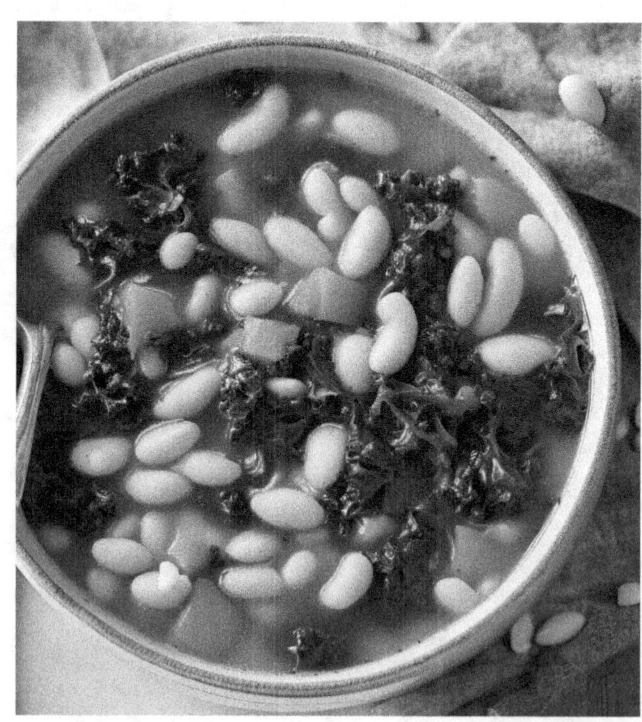

## 20. Fennel and Potato Stew

**Ingredients:**

- 2 tbsp olive oil
- 1 onion, chopped
- 3 garlic cloves, minced
- 2 fennel bulbs, chopped
- 4 potatoes, peeled and diced
- 4 cups vegetable broth (low sodium)
- 1 tsp dried thyme
- 1 bay leaf
- 1 tbsp lemon juice

**Instructions:**

1. Heat olive oil in a large pot over medium heat.
2. Add the onion and garlic, cooking until softened, about 5 minutes.
3. Add the chopped fennel and potatoes, stirring to combine.
4. Pour in the vegetable broth and add the dried thyme and bay leaf. Bring to a boil.
5. Reduce heat and simmer for 25-30 minutes, or until the potatoes are tender.
6. Remove the bay leaf and stir in the lemon juice.
7. Serve hot.

**Nutrition Info (per serving):**

- Calories: 220
- Protein: 4g
- Carbohydrates: 40g
- Fat: 7g
- Fiber: 5g
- Sugar: 6g

**Serves:**

4

**Cooking Time:**

40 minutes

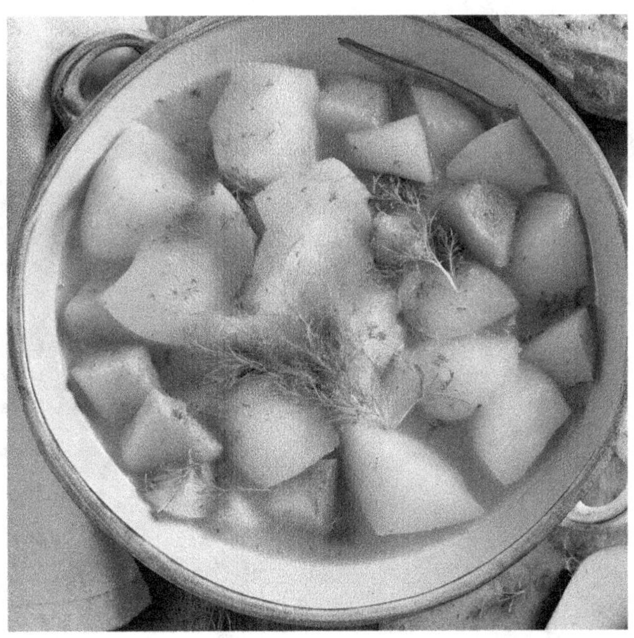

## 21. Green Bean and Almond Soup

**Ingredients:**

- 2 tbsp olive oil
- 1 onion, chopped
- 3 garlic cloves, minced
- 1 lb green beans, trimmed and chopped
- 4 cups vegetable broth (low sodium)
- 1/2 cup almond meal
- 1 cup almond milk
- 1 tbsp lemon juice

**Instructions:**

1. Heat olive oil in a large pot over medium heat.
2. Add the onion and garlic, cooking until softened, about 5 minutes.
3. Add the green beans and cook for another 5 minutes.
4. Pour in the vegetable broth and bring to a boil.
5. Reduce heat and simmer for 15 minutes, or until the green beans are tender.
6. Stir in the almond meal and almond milk, heating through.
7. Blend the soup with an immersion blender or in a regular blender until smooth.
8. Stir in the lemon juice.
9. Serve hot.

**Nutrition Info (per serving):**

- Calories: 180
- Protein: 6g
- Carbohydrates: 14g
- Fat: 12g
- Fiber: 4g
- Sugar: 4g

**Serves:**

4

**Cooking Time:**

30 minutes

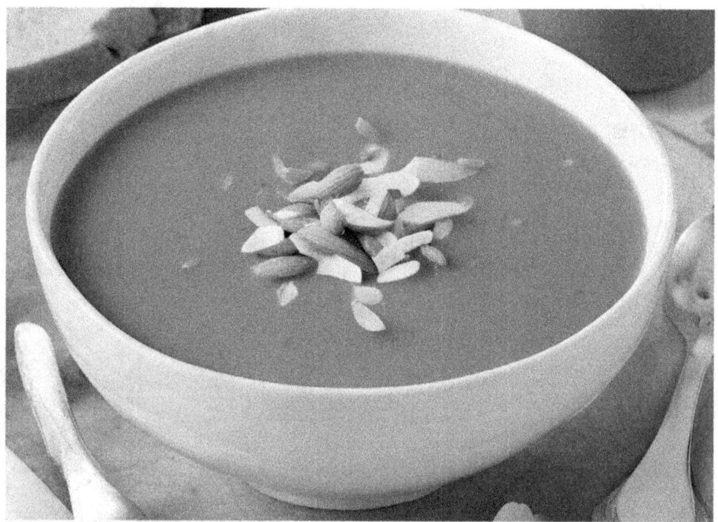

# 8-WEEK MEAL PLAN

## Week 1

**Monday**
- **Breakfast:** Quinoa Porridge
- **Lunch:** Honey Mustard Chicken Salad
- **Dinner:** Baked Chicken with Artichokes and Capers
- **Snack/Dessert:** Almond Yogurt with Kiwi

**Tuesday**
- **Breakfast:** Chia Pudding
- **Lunch:** Turkey Stuffed Mushrooms
- **Dinner:** Tilapia Piccata without Capers
- **Snack/Dessert:** Banana Oat Cookies

**Wednesday**
- **Breakfast:** Oatmeal with Flaxseeds
- **Lunch:** Chicken and Quinoa Salad
- **Dinner:** Moroccan Chicken Tagine
- **Snack/Dessert:** Baked Avocado Eggs

**Thursday**
- **Breakfast:** Buckwheat Pancakes
- **Lunch:** Chicken Vegetable Pot Pie
- **Dinner:** Lemon Tarragon Turkey Cutlets
- **Snack/Dessert:** Berry and Coconut Smoothie

**Friday**
- **Breakfast:** Turmeric Tofu Scramble
- **Lunch:** Asian Turkey Lettuce Cups
- **Dinner:** Pescado Zarandeado (Grilled Snapper)
- **Snack/Dessert:** Pumpkin Seed Granola

**Saturday**
- **Breakfast:** Almond Yogurt with Kiwi
- **Lunch:** Chicken Minestrone Soup
- **Dinner:** Perch with Roasted Almond Slivers
- **Snack/Dessert:** Spirulina Smoothie

**Sunday**
- **Breakfast:** Banana Oat Cookies
- **Lunch:** Chicken Fajitas with Bell Peppers and Onions
- **Dinner:** Shrimp and Spinach Frittata
- **Snack/Dessert:** Grilled Asparagus and Tomato Skewers

## Week 2

**Monday**

- **Breakfast:** Quinoa Porridge
- **Lunch:** Chicken Paillard with Rocket Salad
- **Dinner:** Mussels in Lemongrass Broth
- **Snack/Dessert:** Raspberry Almond Muffins

**Tuesday**

- **Breakfast:** Chia Pudding
- **Lunch:** Chicken Ratatouille
- **Dinner:** Flounder with Parsley and Garlic Butter
- **Snack/Dessert:** Pineapple and Cucumber Salad

**Wednesday**

- **Breakfast:** Oatmeal with Flaxseeds
- **Lunch:** Turkey Bolognese with Zucchini Noodles
- **Dinner:** Swordfish Kebabs with Vegetables
- **Snack/Dessert:** Sweet Potato Muffins

**Thursday**

- **Breakfast:** Buckwheat Pancakes
- **Lunch:** Smoked Salmon and Cucumber Rolls
- **Dinner:** Peppered Mackerel with Salad
- **Snack/Dessert:** Spinach and Mushroom Crepes

**Friday**

- **Breakfast:** Turmeric Tofu Scramble
- **Lunch:** Chicken Ratatouille
- **Dinner:** Moroccan Chickpea Stew
- **Snack/Dessert:** Walnut and Banana Pancakes

**Saturday**

- **Breakfast:** Almond Yogurt with Kiwi
- **Lunch:** Egg Drop Soup
- **Dinner:** Roasted Duck with Orange Sauce
- **Snack/Dessert:** Homemade Seed Bread

**Sunday**

- **Breakfast:** Banana Oat Cookies
- **Lunch:** Beetroot and Ginger Soup
- **Dinner:** Chicken and Broccoli Alfredo
- **Snack/Dessert:** Grilled Asparagus and Tomato Skewers

# Week 3

**Monday**
- **Breakfast:** Quinoa Porridge
- **Lunch:** Bok Choy and Mushroom Soup
- **Dinner:** Haddock Baked with Mustard and Herbs
- **Snack/Dessert:** Pumpkin Seed Granola

**Tuesday**
- **Breakfast:** Chia Pudding
- **Lunch:** Chicken Fajitas with Bell Peppers and Onions
- **Dinner:** Lemon Butter Barramundi
- **Snack/Dessert:** Berry and Coconut Smoothie

**Wednesday**
- **Breakfast:** Oatmeal with Flaxseeds
- **Lunch:** Italian Herb Chicken with Roasted Vegetables
- **Dinner:** Scallop Ceviche with Avocado
- **Snack/Dessert:** Pineapple and Cucumber Salad

**Thursday**
- **Breakfast:** Buckwheat Pancakes
- **Lunch:** Thai Basil Chicken
- **Dinner:** Catfish in Tomato Basil Sauce
- **Snack/Dessert:** Sweet Potato Muffins

**Friday**
- **Breakfast:** Turmeric Tofu Scramble
- **Lunch:** Chicken and Quinoa Salad
- **Dinner:** Chicken Piccata without Capers
- **Snack/Dessert:** Raspberry Almond Muffins

**Saturday**
- **Breakfast:** Almond Yogurt with Kiwi
- **Lunch:** Kale and Potato Soup
- **Dinner:** Perch with Roasted Almond Slivers
- **Snack/Dessert:** Spirulina Smoothie

**Sunday**
- **Breakfast:** Banana Oat Cookies
- **Lunch:** Chicken Minestrone Soup
- **Dinner:** Tilapia Piccata without Capers
- **Snack/Dessert:** Homemade Seed Bread

## Week 4

**Monday**
- **Breakfast:** Quinoa Porridge
- **Lunch:** Chicken Paillard with Rocket Salad
- **Dinner:** Kingfish Sashimi with Soy and Wasabi
- **Snack/Dessert:** Spinach and Mushroom Crepes

**Tuesday**
- **Breakfast:** Chia Pudding
- **Lunch:** Shrimp and Spinach Frittata
- **Dinner:** Prawn Stir-Fry with Broccoli and Bell Peppers
- **Snack/Dessert:** Pineapple and Cucumber Salad

**Wednesday**
- **Breakfast:** Oatmeal with Flaxseeds
- **Lunch:** Chicken Ratatouille
- **Dinner:** Grilled Trout with Herbs
- **Snack/Dessert:** Raspberry Almond Muffins

**Thursday**
- **Breakfast:** Buckwheat Pancakes
- **Lunch:** Chicken Fajitas with Bell Peppers and Onions
- **Dinner:** Sweet Potato and Black Bean Chili
- **Snack/Dessert:** Sweet Potato Muffins

**Friday**
- **Breakfast:** Turmeric Tofu Scramble
- **Lunch:** Celery Soup
- **Dinner:** Sardines Grilled with Lemon Pepper
- **Snack/Dessert:** Spirulina Smoothie

**Saturday**
- **Breakfast:** Almond Yogurt with Kiwi
- **Lunch:** Italian White Bean and Kale Soup
- **Dinner:** Roasted Turkey Breast with Rosemary and Sage
- **Snack/Dessert:** Walnut and Banana Pancakes

**Sunday**
- **Breakfast:** Banana Oat Cookies
- **Lunch:** Zucchini Soup
- **Dinner:** Lobster Tail Steamed with Ginger
- **Snack/Dessert:** Grilled Asparagus and Tomato Skewers

# Week 5

**Monday**
- **Breakfast:** Vegetable Omelette
- **Lunch:** Broccoli Almond Soup
- **Dinner:** Moroccan Chicken Tagine
- **Snack/Dessert:** Baked Avocado Eggs

**Tuesday**
- **Breakfast:** Zucchini Muffins
- **Lunch:** Spicy Tomato and Lentil Soup
- **Dinner:** Lemon Tarragon Turkey Cutlets
- **Snack/Dessert:** Berry and Coconut Smoothie

**Wednesday**
- **Breakfast:** Fruit Salad
- **Lunch:** Split Pea Soup
- **Dinner:** Smoked Paprika Chicken Thighs
- **Snack/Dessert:** Sweet Potato Muffins

**Thursday**
- **Breakfast:** Sautéed Kale and Mushrooms
- **Lunch:** Carrot Ginger Soup
- **Dinner:** Tilapia Piccata without Capers
- **Snack/Dessert:** Spirulina Smoothie

**Friday**
- **Breakfast:** Banana Oat Cookies
- **Lunch:** Chicken Fajitas with Bell Peppers and Onions
- **Dinner:** Thai Coconut Shrimp Soup
- **Snack/Dessert:** Raspberry Almond Muffins

**Saturday**
- **Breakfast:** Turmeric Tofu Scramble
- **Lunch:** Fennel and Potato Stew
- **Dinner:** Grilled Trout with Herbs
- **Snack/Dessert:** Homemade Seed Bread

**Sunday**
- **Breakfast:** Buckwheat Pancakes
- **Lunch:** Beetroot and Ginger Soup
- **Dinner:** Chicken and Broccoli Alfredo
- **Snack/Dessert:** Pineapple and Cucumber Salad

# Week 6

**Monday**
- **Breakfast:** Almond Yogurt with Kiwi
- **Lunch:** Bok Choy and Mushroom Soup
- **Dinner:** Lemon Butter Barramundi
- **Snack/Dessert:** Spinach and Mushroom Crepes

**Tuesday**
- **Breakfast:** Quinoa Porridge
- **Lunch:** Sweet Potato and Black Bean Chili
- **Dinner:** Perch with Roasted Almond Slivers
- **Snack/Dessert:** Berry and Coconut Smoothie

**Wednesday**
- **Breakfast:** Chia Pudding
- **Lunch:** Chicken Minestrone Soup
- **Dinner:** Prawn Stir-Fry with Broccoli and Bell Peppers
- **Snack/Dessert:** Raspberry Almond Muffins

**Thursday**
- **Breakfast:** Oatmeal with Flaxseeds
- **Lunch:** Zucchini Soup
- **Dinner:** Scallop Ceviche with Avocado
- **Snack/Dessert:** Spirulina Smoothie

**Friday**
- **Breakfast:** Buckwheat Pancakes
- **Lunch:** Kale and Potato Soup
- **Dinner:** Chicken Piccata without Capers
- **Snack/Dessert:** Pineapple and Cucumber Salad

**Saturday**
- **Breakfast:** Turmeric Tofu Scramble
- **Lunch:** Fennel and Potato Stew
- **Dinner:** Moroccan Chickpea Stew
- **Snack/Dessert:** Sweet Potato Muffins

**Sunday**
- **Breakfast:** Banana Oat Cookies
- **Lunch:** Green Bean and Almond Soup
- **Dinner:** Roasted Duck with Orange Sauce
- **Snack/Dessert:** Homemade Seed Bread

# Week 7

**Monday**
- **Breakfast:** Vegetable Omelette
- **Lunch:** Spicy Tomato and Lentil Soup
- **Dinner:** Smoked Paprika Chicken Thighs
- **Snack/Dessert:** Baked Avocado Eggs

**Tuesday**
- **Breakfast:** Zucchini Muffins
- **Lunch:** Celery Soup
- **Dinner:** Lemon Tarragon Turkey Cutlets
- **Snack/Dessert:** Berry and Coconut Smoothie

**Wednesday**
- **Breakfast:** Fruit Salad
- **Lunch:** Split Pea Soup
- **Dinner:** Tilapia Piccata without Capers
- **Snack/Dessert:** Sweet Potato Muffins

**Thursday**
- **Breakfast:** Sautéed Kale and Mushrooms
- **Lunch:** Carrot Ginger Soup
- **Dinner:** Chicken Piccata without Capers
- **Snack/Dessert:** Spirulina Smoothie

**Friday**
- **Breakfast:** Banana Oat Cookies
- **Lunch:** Chicken Fajitas with Bell Peppers and Onions
- **Dinner:** Thai Coconut Shrimp Soup
- **Snack/Dessert:** Raspberry Almond Muffins

**Saturday**
- **Breakfast:** Turmeric Tofu Scramble
- **Lunch:** Bok Choy and Mushroom Soup
- **Dinner:** Grilled Trout with Herbs
- **Snack/Dessert:** Homemade Seed Bread

**Sunday**
- **Breakfast:** Buckwheat Pancakes
- **Lunch:** Beetroot and Ginger Soup
- **Dinner:** Chicken and Broccoli Alfredo
- **Snack/Dessert:** Pineapple and Cucumber Salad

## Week 8

**Monday**
- **Breakfast:** Almond Yogurt with Kiwi
- **Lunch:** Sweet Potato and Black Bean Chili
- **Dinner:** Perch with Roasted Almond Slivers
- **Snack/Dessert:** Spinach and Mushroom Crepes

**Tuesday**
- **Breakfast:** Quinoa Porridge
- **Lunch:** Chicken Minestrone Soup
- **Dinner:** Lemon Butter Barramundi
- **Snack/Dessert:** Berry and Coconut Smoothie

**Wednesday**
- **Breakfast:** Chia Pudding
- **Lunch:** Zucchini Soup
- **Dinner:** Prawn Stir-Fry with Broccoli and Bell Peppers
- **Snack/Dessert:** Raspberry Almond Muffins

**Thursday**
- **Breakfast:** Oatmeal with Flaxseeds
- **Lunch:** Kale and Potato Soup
- **Dinner:** Scallop Ceviche with Avocado
- **Snack/Dessert:** Spirulina Smoothie

**Friday**
- **Breakfast:** Buckwheat Pancakes
- **Lunch:** Fennel and Potato Stew
- **Dinner:** Chicken Piccata without Capers
- **Snack/Dessert:** Pineapple and Cucumber Salad

**Saturday**
- **Breakfast:** Turmeric Tofu Scramble
- **Lunch:** Green Bean and Almond Soup
- **Dinner:** Moroccan Chickpea Stew
- **Snack/Dessert:** Sweet Potato Muffins

**Sunday**
- **Breakfast:** Banana Oat Cookies
- **Lunch:** Carrot Ginger Soup
- **Dinner:** Roasted Duck with Orange Sauce
- **Snack/Dessert:** Homemade Seed Bread

# WEEKLY MEAL PLANNER + WORKBOOK

|  | BREAKFAST | LUNCH | DINNER | SNACKS |
|---|---|---|---|---|
| MONDAY |  |  |  |  |
| TUESDAY |  |  |  |  |
| WEDNESDAY |  |  |  |  |
| THURSDAY |  |  |  |  |
| FRIDAY |  |  |  |  |
| SATURDAY |  |  |  |  |
| SUNDAY |  |  |  |  |

**WHAT ARE YOUR CURRENT ENDOMETRIOSIS SYMPTOMS, AND HOW SEVERE ARE THEY ON A SCALE OF 1-10?**

# WEEKLY MEAL PLANNER + WORKBOOK

|  | BREAKFAST | LUNCH | DINNER | SNACKS |
|---|---|---|---|---|
| MONDAY | | | | |
| TUESDAY | | | | |
| WEDNESDAY | | | | |
| THURSDAY | | | | |
| FRIDAY | | | | |
| SATURDAY | | | | |
| SUNDAY | | | | |

**WHAT DOES A TYPICAL DAY'S MEALS LOOK LIKE FOR YOU? INCLUDE BREAKFAST, LUNCH, DINNER, AND SNACKS.**

# WEEKLY MEAL PLANNER + WORKBOOK

| | BREAKFAST | LUNCH | DINNER | SNACKS |
|---|---|---|---|---|
| MONDAY | | | | |
| TUESDAY | | | | |
| WEDNESDAY | | | | |
| THURSDAY | | | | |
| FRIDAY | | | | |
| SATURDAY | | | | |
| SUNDAY | | | | |

**WHAT ARE YOUR PRIMARY GOALS FOR STARTING THE ENDOMETRIOSIS DIET? (E.G., PAIN REDUCTION, INCREASED ENERGY, WEIGHT MANAGEMENT)**

# WEEKLY MEAL PLANNER + WORKBOOK

|  | BREAKFAST | LUNCH | DINNER | SNACKS |
|---|---|---|---|---|
| MONDAY |  |  |  |  |
| TUESDAY |  |  |  |  |
| WEDNESDAY |  |  |  |  |
| THURSDAY |  |  |  |  |
| FRIDAY |  |  |  |  |
| SATURDAY |  |  |  |  |
| SUNDAY |  |  |  |  |

**HAVE YOU NOTICED ANY CHANGES IN YOUR SYMPTOMS AFTER THE FIRST WEEK OF FOLLOWING THE DIET? DESCRIBE THEM.**

# WEEKLY MEAL PLANNER + WORKBOOK

|  | BREAKFAST | LUNCH | DINNER | SNACKS |
|---|---|---|---|---|
| MONDAY |  |  |  |  |
| TUESDAY |  |  |  |  |
| WEDNESDAY |  |  |  |  |
| THURSDAY |  |  |  |  |
| FRIDAY |  |  |  |  |
| SATURDAY |  |  |  |  |
| SUNDAY |  |  |  |  |

**HOW DO YOU FEEL EMOTIONALLY ABOUT THE DIETARY CHANGES YOU HAVE MADE SO FAR? (E.G., EXCITED, OVERWHELMED, HOPEFUL)**

.......................................................................................................................................

.......................................................................................................................................

.......................................................................................................................................

.......................................................................................................................................

.......................................................................................................................................

.......................................................................................................................................

# WEEKLY MEAL PLANNER + WORKBOOK

|  | BREAKFAST | LUNCH | DINNER | SNACKS |
|---|---|---|---|---|
| MONDAY |  |  |  |  |
| TUESDAY |  |  |  |  |
| WEDNESDAY |  |  |  |  |
| THURSDAY |  |  |  |  |
| FRIDAY |  |  |  |  |
| SATURDAY |  |  |  |  |
| SUNDAY |  |  |  |  |

**HAVE YOU EXPERIENCED ANY SYMPTOM FLARE-UPS? IF SO, WHAT DID YOU EAT THAT DAY?**

# WEEKLY MEAL PLANNER + WORKBOOK

| | BREAKFAST | LUNCH | DINNER | SNACKS |
|---|---|---|---|---|
| MONDAY | | | | |
| TUESDAY | | | | |
| WEDNESDAY | | | | |
| THURSDAY | | | | |
| FRIDAY | | | | |
| SATURDAY | | | | |
| SUNDAY | | | | |

**WHICH MEALS FROM THE ENDOMETRIOSIS DIET HAVE YOU ENJOYED THE MOST? WHY?**

# WEEKLY MEAL PLANNER + WORKBOOK

|  | BREAKFAST | LUNCH | DINNER | SNACKS |
|---|---|---|---|---|
| MONDAY | | | | |
| TUESDAY | | | | |
| WEDNESDAY | | | | |
| THURSDAY | | | | |
| FRIDAY | | | | |
| SATURDAY | | | | |
| SUNDAY | | | | |

**WHAT CHALLENGES HAVE YOU FACED WHILE FOLLOWING THE DIET, AND HOW HAVE YOU OVERCOME THEM?**

# WEEKLY MEAL PLANNER + WORKBOOK

| | BREAKFAST | LUNCH | DINNER | SNACKS |
|---|---|---|---|---|
| MONDAY | | | | |
| TUESDAY | | | | |
| WEDNESDAY | | | | |
| THURSDAY | | | | |
| FRIDAY | | | | |
| SATURDAY | | | | |
| SUNDAY | | | | |

**WHAT ADJUSTMENTS HAVE YOU MADE TO THE DIET TO BETTER SUIT YOUR PREFERENCES AND LIFESTYLE?**

# WEEKLY MEAL PLANNER + WORKBOOK

|  | BREAKFAST | LUNCH | DINNER | SNACKS |
|---|---|---|---|---|
| MONDAY | | | | |
| TUESDAY | | | | |
| WEDNESDAY | | | | |
| THURSDAY | | | | |
| FRIDAY | | | | |
| SATURDAY | | | | |
| SUNDAY | | | | |

**HOW HAVE YOUR ENERGY LEVELS CHANGED SINCE STARTING THE DIET? PROVIDE SPECIFIC EXAMPLES.**

# WEEKLY MEAL PLANNER + WORKBOOK

|  | BREAKFAST | LUNCH | DINNER | SNACKS |
|---|---|---|---|---|
| MONDAY |  |  |  |  |
| TUESDAY |  |  |  |  |
| WEDNESDAY |  |  |  |  |
| THURSDAY |  |  |  |  |
| FRIDAY |  |  |  |  |
| SATURDAY |  |  |  |  |
| SUNDAY |  |  |  |  |

**HOW HAS YOUR GROCERY SHOPPING LIST CHANGED SINCE YOU STARTED THE DIET? LIST SOME NEW STAPLES YOU'VE ADDED.**

# WEEKLY MEAL PLANNER + WORKBOOK

|  | BREAKFAST | LUNCH | DINNER | SNACKS |
|---|---|---|---|---|
| MONDAY | | | | |
| TUESDAY | | | | |
| WEDNESDAY | | | | |
| THURSDAY | | | | |
| FRIDAY | | | | |
| SATURDAY | | | | |
| SUNDAY | | | | |

**HAVE YOU DEVELOPED ANY NEW ROUTINES OR HABITS AS A RESULT OF FOLLOWING THE DIET? DESCRIBE THEM.**

# WEEKLY MEAL PLANNER  +  WORKBOOK

|  | BREAKFAST | LUNCH | DINNER | SNACKS |
|---|---|---|---|---|
| MONDAY | | | | |
| TUESDAY | | | | |
| WEDNESDAY | | | | |
| THURSDAY | | | | |
| FRIDAY | | | | |
| SATURDAY | | | | |
| SUNDAY | | | | |

**WHO IN YOUR LIFE HAS BEEN SUPPORTIVE OF YOUR DIETARY CHANGES? HOW HAVE THEY SUPPORTED YOU?**

# WEEKLY MEAL PLANNER + WORKBOOK

| | BREAKFAST | LUNCH | DINNER | SNACKS |
|---|---|---|---|---|
| MONDAY | | | | |
| TUESDAY | | | | |
| WEDNESDAY | | | | |
| THURSDAY | | | | |
| FRIDAY | | | | |
| SATURDAY | | | | |
| SUNDAY | | | | |

**WHAT LONG-TERM HEALTH GOALS DO YOU HAVE NOW THAT YOU'VE BEEN FOLLOWING THE ENDOMETRIOSIS DIET FOR SEVERAL WEEKS?**

# WEEKLY MEAL PLANNER + WORKBOOK

|  | BREAKFAST | LUNCH | DINNER | SNACKS |
|---|---|---|---|---|
| MONDAY | | | | |
| TUESDAY | | | | |
| WEDNESDAY | | | | |
| THURSDAY | | | | |
| FRIDAY | | | | |
| SATURDAY | | | | |
| SUNDAY | | | | |

**WHAT ADVICE WOULD YOU GIVE TO SOMEONE WHO IS JUST STARTING THE ENDOMETRIOSIS DIET?**

# Scan the QR code below to get a surprise bonus!

www.ingramcontent.com/pod-product-compliance
Lightning Source LLC
Chambersburg PA
CBHW081517250726
48659CB00009B/2841